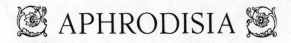

# APHRODISIA

*A Guide to*
Herbs

APHRO

GARY

A DUTTON

E. P. DUTTON

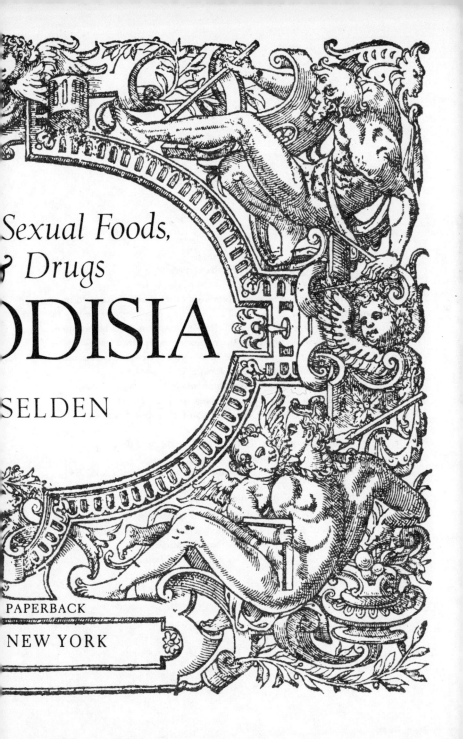

*Sexual Foods,*
*& Drugs*

ODISIA

SELDEN

PAPERBACK

NEW YORK

For information contact:
E. P. Dutton, 2 Park Avenue, New York, N.Y.   10016
Library of Congress Cataloging in Publication Data
Selden, Gary.
Aphrodisia: a guide to sexual food, herbs, and drugs.
Bibliography: p. 227
1.Food.   2.Herbs.   3.Drugs.   4.Aphrodisiacs.   I.Title.   TX357.S44
1979   615′.766   79-10671
ISBN: 0-525-47594-X
Published simultaneously in Canada by
Clarke, Irwin & Company Limited, Toronto and Vancouver
Designed by Barbara Huntley
10 9 8 7 6 5 4 3 2 1   First Edition

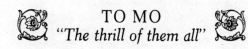

TO MO
*"The thrill of them all"*

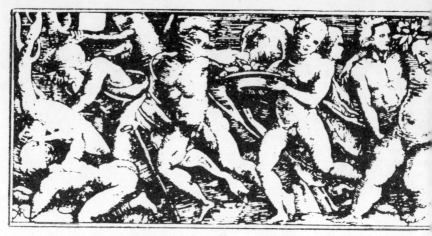

# Contents

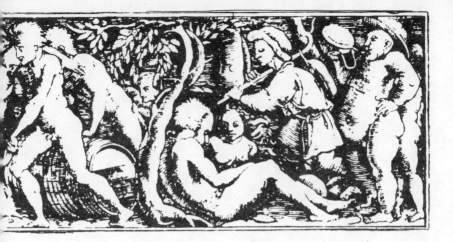

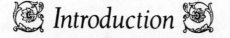# Introduction

LET'S say you're with your lover watching the inevitable prese-duction dinner in some spy flick, or maybe *Tom Jones* for the umpteenth time. Up there on the screen are the exaggerated mouthings on the drumstick, the winks, the sighing sidelong glances, the dangling conversations, and the quick dilation and contraction of the iris that shows Cupid's arrow got them right in the eye. Grapes in hand, she brushes his ankle, then his thigh, with her foot. In the audience your companion slips a hand into your crotch, and suddenly, in a fanfare of silent trumpets, you're lost in a fantasy of your own. Couples and small groups are seen in other corners of the movie dining room; new vistas open through a window where a garden orgy is in full tilt.

A fountain spouting wine instead of water bathes three or four naked couples who splash in it like hot-blooded fish at spawning season. A man covered with peanut butter and a woman spread with jelly sandwich themselves together between halves of an enormous French bread. A sailor wearing only his hat sails away with a mermaid waist-deep in a vat of oysters. Another uni-dentifiable couple lick the whipped cream off each other as fast as they can spread it on. A palomino blonde covered from head to foot with honey slithers back and forth between two sticky lovers.

In the center of the spectacle is a huge doughnut-shaped table. Within the hole a maître d' directs the parade of food being brought up from the underground galley. Just as a bowl of caviar emerges, an obstreperous, curly-headed wench seizes a blue-eyed bloke's hair and plunges his face into it, then climbs up around his waist and licks roe from his cheeks between giggles. Cossets, custards, cornucopias of shining fruit, tureens of turtle soup, platters of fish, and plates of asparagus stream from the innards of this magic table. Bananas and pickles are tenderly wielded. A tall brunette lasciviously accepts her admirer's proffered pepperoni. A pixie has a red-bearded giant nearly covered with cinnamon frosting when he carries her over one arm to a nearby bed of marshmallows. Peaches roll down the marble pathways into a pool of pomegranate juice. Dazed and flushed, you and your lover hurriedly leave the theater for the nearest bedroom.

Food and lovemaking have gone together at orgies and seduction dinners for ages, and yet when the subject of aphrodisiacs comes up, one question never fails to arise: "Do they really exist?" Before this or its follow-up, "Could you get me some?" can be answered, a flotilla of implied assumptions and preconceptions must be examined.

Even after a decade of Aquarianism, we are a stiff-necked, methodical people, true to our rationalist forebears and in awe of our priestly scientists. For every conclusion we demand reams of statistics and double-blind experiments yielding charts and graphs. To believe in aphrodisiacs we need a purified extract that we can tipple at our leisure, its label endorsed with grateful testimonials. We know all about Freud and his cigars; we know what invariably follows the adjective "melon-shaped." Still, we usually miss the connection that our very language charts for us across the intimate geography of food and sex.

A conversation is meaningless unless its participants agree on the meanings of the words they use. Since "aphrodisiac" has included so many different definitions, we had better clarify. At its broadest, the word takes in any stimulus that sexually excites *anybody*. That can mean beautiful women, beautiful men, clothing, nudity, baths, body odor, perfumes, massage, whippings, feasts, flowers, music, movies, satin sheets, and all the rest. A preliminary distinction is usually drawn between internal aphrodisiacs, like foods and drugs, and external or collateral aphrodisiacs, like unguents, apparel, scents, and visions of loveliness. Even so, it can be hard, as in the case of the dildo, to differentiate completely.

It is mainly the internal aphrodisiacs we'll be considering, but even this term encompasses too much. Its definition is a catalog of the sexual improvements people want. An internal aphrodisiac is anything swallowed that: increases sensual awareness in the genitals or throughout the body, makes erections easier and harder, promotes clitoral excitation and vaginal secretion, stimulates genital nerves, promotes domestic tranquility, releases inhibitions, increases semen production, prevents abrupt ejaculation, lessens the psychological or physical causes of impotence or frigidity, prevents or reverses the sexual deterioration caused by aging, replenishes the body after exhaustion, energizes mind or body, strengthens the emotions, or gradually tones glands. It's no wonder there are a lot of aphrodisiacs. (It's too bad that the word, aphrodisiac, with that horrible "ack" at the end, is so *an*aphrodisiac. Aphrodisia, the state of being there, is more euphonious, but we sorely need a short, sweet synonym for our subject. An aphro? A dizzy? An erotizer? A cupidor?)

What we lack in words we can make up for in examples. Besides the entries that follow, various lovers have put their faith in horseradish, tripe, bat's blood, dried salamanders, prunes, tulip bulbs, camel's hump fat, bee's wings, crushed crickets and dragonflies, valerian root, toad bones, and *aquae amatrices* (the water of sulfurous springs).

Judging from folklore, there is almost nothing we can eat (except too much of a good thing) that *isn't* an aphrodisiac. Nearly every known food and each of many hundreds of herbs have a reputation somewhere in the world for inciting lust. The "problem" is that in the right frame of mind, with a congenial partner, *anything* will work to perfection, producing hard proof of the prescription's effectiveness. So we see that science here is on a footing—or bedding—altogether different from its research posture in other fields.

The food-love connection is physiological from the start. The moist, delicate mouth shares many traits with the other moist, delicate areas to the south. One of the most telling is the location of Krause's end-bulbs, the unusually large and sensitive nerve endings that are concentrated in the penis or clitoris and . . . the lips. Many biological comparisons have likewise been drawn between the taste buds and the heads of the erectile organs. Sexual tension and the smell of food can both make the mouth water (though lust can also dry it out momentarily). The nutritive and amative drives merge into bliss during a kiss, that quaint mammalian custom in which a taste leads to the satisfaction of hunger. Oral-genital amour may result primarily from the yearning to unite our two regions of Krause's bulbs. And every day millions of hickeys, peering over the tops of shirt collars or lurking in more secluded spots, show that the line between screwing and chewing is easily crossed.

Copulation has often been described as a function of the digestive system, because it cannot occur to the fullest—or sometimes at all—if the body is malnourished. We all know the languid euphoria that follows an ample, creatively cooked meal, served with piquant sauces and a fine wine. This state of satiety and contentment conduces to venery more than most other moods, and it leads us to the first type of aphrodisiac we are seeking. We want to know what foods, what diet, what balance of nutrient and exercise will keep us in the best possible shape to enjoy our love lives. What foods best promote secretion of hormones, semen, and vaginal juices? How does one construct the perfect prelude meal, wherein sight, smell, taste, texture, and vitamins all conspire to send us frenzied to the threshing floor of love? We must test those nutrition concentrates born of the health-food industry and likewise try the recipes of antiquity.

Few still think that life must be the sexless proving ground for heaven that the Puritans made it. The related notion that rational folk must rise above their animal desires is also being abandoned. But in the aftermath of Victorianism many people applied the test ethic to sex. Even today many sexologists make lovemaking sound like weight lifting, with their incessant talk of the proper "regimen" for "optimum performance" of "the act." But our lives are a sort of training nonetheless, with recurrent workouts and rests. And without making it too much of a duty, shouldn't we train most eagerly for the most rewarding game? Eating and loving can lead us to the kind of practical religion that Vatsyayana sought in his "Love Text," or *Kama Sutra*—for, according to Hindu teaching, *kama* (love/sex/pleasure) is the womb of *artha* (achievement) and *dharma* (virtue), and it is the right mixture of the three that makes human life a joy to lead.

With this end in mind, we must next try to separate the biological effects of the foods and herbs from the psychological effects of their physical shape or reputation. Two concepts must now be sorted out, one ancient, one modern.

The Doctrine of Signatures, a belief current since an unknown prehistoric date, maintains that all life on earth is held in a network of affinities that various life-forms have for each other. It teaches that the use of a plant or animal can be known by the resemblance of some part of it to the human organ it can aid. In other words, like cures like. Oysters are good for the testicles because God made them look like testicles, and mandrake helps women make babies because its bifurcated root often looks like a little human. Because this belief sounds so patently silly to our literal, logically trained minds, many are quick to say that all reputed aphrodisiacs are imaginary. As we shall see, scientific confirmation of many such beliefs suggests that the doctrine, although sometimes a guide to theobotanical fantasy, was primarily a mnemonic aid to plant lore already tested by experience.

We must also account for a newer doctrine, the Placebo Factor. Its name derives from medical tests in which an experimental drug is given randomly to some patients while an inert substance, or placebo, is given to others. Neither the experimenters nor the subjects know beforehand who is getting the real thing. Depending on the disease involved, about 20 to 30 percent of those who draw the blanks will show an improvement anyway, demonstrating the power of mind over malaise. Current theory suggests that the expectation of aid causes the brain more effectively to marshal the body's disease defenses and pain-relieving endorphins (internal opiates).

In any endeavor as filled with nuances of confidence as love, the placebo factor can well be the deciding one. How many spells were intended solely to screw the power of expectation to its highest pitch? Even in these realistic times there are people who are said to be able to levitate, bend forks, or otherwise change solid objects with their minds alone. Why might such concentration not affect something so vaporous and changeable as our own passions, or someone else's? Perhaps we will have to consider a Magic Factor in our calculations. Since sex itself can *be* magic, and since both work by charms, this should hardly surprise us.

Philippa Pullar, in her *Consuming Passions,** a curious study of sexuality and English cuisine, traces the belief in aphrodisiacs to animistic religions in which a spirit presided over every object and abstraction in the universe. Thus sexual arousal was an invisible force that came from outside the bodies of the people involved. It could be triggered or released only by invoking the

* For complete reference information for this and other works cited in the text, see Selected Bibliography, pages 227–231.

presiding deity and perhaps aiding its work by its favorite plant, animal, or stone. Although this is too simplistic a view of ancient faiths, many people in all ages have lived at this level of superstition, and we must expect much aphrodisiac folklore to be nothing but religious rumors amplified by time. From the historical heyday of aphrodisiacs—in the cultures of Egypt, the Near East, Greece, and Rome—precious little detail survives. Much was never written down so that jealous love doctors could guard their best recipes, and much that was written was destroyed by the zealous Church, eager to suppress the sexual center of pagan sin.

The uncertainty of legend produces the characteristic style of books on aphrodisiacs. The such-and-such fruit "is said to be" a remedy for impotence, or the root of the never-never bush "reputedly" enabled the Duke of Hasbeenshire to deflower a hundred virgins in one night. Moreover, the Gullibility Component was especially profitable to explorers when travel was rare and arduous. Many a tale was embellished with fabled trees, their lustful seed pods, and the lost secrets of the ancients found anew. Potions concocted of baser ingredients were regularly palmed off on the folks back home. Donizetti's opera *L'Elisir d'Amore* is built around this timeless hustle. The prescription of Dr. Dulcamara ("Bittersweet"), purportedly the lost recipe of Tristan and Isolde, is but wine. It works, though: the exorbitant price instills faith in it, and the doctor's advice—chase and you'll be fled, flee and you'll be followed—actually does get Nemorino and Adina together at last.

The elixir of money alone is a potent aphrodisiac. Exotic and erotic are only one letter apart. Rarity creates demand, demand creates price, and every ingestible with an outrageous price is legendary in the bedroom. This relation applies equally to cocaine, truffles, pâté de foie gras, pearls in wine, rhinoceros horn, and caviar, whatever their physiological virtues. When they were still half a world away, the spices of the Indies were considered surefire aphrodisiacs. This law of rarity is best exemplified by the potato. When *Solanum tuberosum* first reached Elizabethan England from the New World, its scarcity gave it a scandalous reputation. In *The Loyal Subject*, John Fletcher asks: "Will your lordship please to taste a fine potato? 'Twill advance your withered state, fill your honor with noble itches." And Shakespeare, using current slang for a penis or dildo, in *Troilus and Cressida* wags "the potato-finger of the devil luxury." But nowadays most people would agree there is no vegetable less venereous than the lowly spud. We must therefore be prepared to find some blind alleys in our search, and to be critical of the naïve enthusiasms of our own time.

It may be that the best aphrodisiacs have been forgotten as our farm system has moved from cultivation of a wide variety of locally grown plants and animals to mass production of fewer, more standardized foods. Better trade networks have no doubt offset some regional limitations—providing oranges to Norway, for example—but the loss of agricultural diversity may have been too high a price to pay. Our abstract harvests of juiceless tomatoes and denutrified "enriched" bread do not encourage us to savor their sexual effects (if any are left).

World distribution of formerly rare edibles and the boredom of habitual use may have changed our reactions so that what used to excite us no longer does. When first introduced to Europe, cocoa was an aphrodisiac so strong it was forbidden to nuns and damned from pulpits, but who today gets laid by offering a Hershey bar? A similar attenuation of response seems to have happened with tea and coffee, and may be occurring today with marijuana and cocaine. Let us hope the elixirs we seek are not extinct, gone the way of the dodo before the onslaught of progress.

No matter what miraculous potions we discover, they will certainly work better at some times than others. Biologists are just beginning to unravel the secrets of inner human rhythm. Many believe in the rigid 23-, 28-, and 33-day cycles popularly known as biorhythms; despite continuing controversy over their validity, they have been successfully used by bus companies and industrial firms to lower worker accident rates. But they are certainly not the only cycles that affect us. The female menstrual cycle is the best known, used for ages as proof of woman's inherent "instability." But lo and behold, men are now known to undergo similar hormone fluctuations that affect mood, mental acuity, and other aspects of life. And all of us show an individual daily rhythm whereby our temperature, pulse, and metabolic activity fluctuate.

Research is still in the early stages, but it is becoming increasingly evident that our lives, including our sex lives, are a symphony of enmeshed cycles that constantly react with or against each other. We have not the space to delve further into the topic here; anyone curious about sexual cycles can get a good start by consulting *Biorhythms and Human Reproduction*. Even without an interest in biorhythm, the thoughtful reader will benefit from the book's introductory essay on the chimerical nature of time. Our point here is simply that no aphrodisiac has an absolute effect; it is always modified by the condition of the lover at the time.

With these cautions in mind, let us try for a clearer idea of what we hope to find. Restorative foods have already been mentioned. But tradition also touts thousands of herbs and spices, with their aromatic oils or alkaloids. The fragrance itself is often said to be enough, but most of these plants also have some effect on our bodies or brains. Among those with the hottest reputation are the pepper plants. Their oils irritate the anus, bladder, and urethra, and by proximity are supposed to heat the gonads as well. Though not a pepper, the cantharides beetle, or Spanish fly, is the best known of these burning products. But the erections it produces are more akin to the excruciating itch of leprosy than the promptings of Priapus. It is too hard to regulate the dose, too painful, and too often fatal to be called an aphrodisiac. Although far more benign, peppers, unless they can be shown to have some direct effect on sexual organs, also must be considered a near-miss.

All substances that release energy in body or mind—such as ginseng, cocaine, cocoa, or tea—are sometimes called aphrodisiacs, though the energy they release can as easily be directed to scrubbing the floor. We are seeking something more directly erotic than any of these. At its heart, the search for aphrodisiacs is a search for external supplements for the internal hormones that govern arousal, perhaps even a chemical that will trip the brain's sexual responses. Here we will settle for a tonic, a daily dose to gradually raise our eroticability level. But the horny grail of our agelong hunt is a potion as sudden and invincible as sex itself, a medicine that without fail will rev up the engine as soon as we swallow it, and keep the throttle wide open for hours before we run out of gas.

The widespread popularity of sex should make aphrodisia one of the most talked-about subjects in the world, but—not counting men's room jokes about Spanish fly—it is rarely discussed. It has long been assumed that the discoverer of a reliable love potion could buy an Arab sheikdom with the proceeds, yet today's marketplace has little to offer but sex-appeal toothpastes and capsules of cayenne advertised as "genuine ersatz Spanish fly" in the back pages of grade D skin magazines. Except for tests on a few hormones and drugs to overcome impotence or frigidity, no modern scientist has ever investigated the topic, despite scores of promising leads and thousands of untested plants.

In fact, we know *less* about aphrodisiacs today than our ancestors did. Throughout the world there once existed an extensive folklore of foods and herbs to fortify the sexual organs, and it is unreasonable to believe that all of it was bogus. Restorative cuisine—nutrient-rich, concentrated, easily digested food chosen for optimum sexual health—was once part of humanity's common knowledge. A few generations of antisexual morality and education have nearly erased these traditions from the West. Marxism, with its Victorian origins and denigration of noncommunal pleasures, has done a similar job in much of the East, although recent wall posters denouncing sexual repression as *anti*socialist bring hope of an awakening in China. The poverty of overpopulation and colonialism has made sex a low-priority concern for many, and the worldwide spread of the processed-food industry threatens to create a species of gastronomical moron who can't imagine a *healthy* meal—much less a sexy one.

A knowledge of aphrodisiacs is both essential and supremely unimportant. It can rescue the nervous, bolster the weak, entertain the healthy, and vividly show the connection between our own sexuality and that of other beings. It can sometimes help the average man approach the greater sexual capacity of the average woman, fostering harmony between the sexes by way of equal satisfaction.

But no aphrodisiac can substitute for health. Not even the stimulative foods can be relied on as a crutch or overused with impunity. Some of the herbs or drugs may help dispel daily cares or the fears resulting from an antisexual upbringing, but when they are relied on too often, unwanted side effects generally appear. None will for long mask the effects of poor diet, lack of exercise and imagination, or boredom with one's mate. After advising the aging Louis XV not to use aphrodisiacs because of his waning health, the king's physician warned of "the greatest aphrodisiac of all"—change. Whether by variety of partners or variety of style, one can have a phenomenal sex life with nothing but a lover. Pietro Aretino quotes the Roman heroine Lucretia as claiming, "The sole philtre that ever I used was kissing and embracing, by which alone I made men rave like beasts stupefied, and compelled them to worship me like an idol."

Still, aphrodisia is like a string of pearls with a black evening dress, a small part of the repertoire of ecstatic refinements dreamed up by eons of lovers, without which the effect of the whole would be greatly diminished. Our sexual civilization has gone underground for centuries and is just beginning to reemerge from the world war waged against it by unworldly religions and sexless lawmakers.

Let us pause here to remember a few of this war's victims.

Besides the millions tortured or killed for witchcraft, fellatio, or coitus without a permit, there were the "surprising number of husbands," patients at Masters and Johnson's clinic, who had never seen their wives' genitals. There were the eighteen wives, reported in Robert Dickinson's early study, *A Thousand Marriages*, who remained virgins after marriage "because neither husband nor wife knew how to perform sexual intercourse." There were the unknown number who never made love except through a *chemise cagoule*, a full-length canvas shroud with one hole just big enough to permit procreation without further damning contact of skin. Among all our statues of Charlemagne, Tamerlane, Pope John, and Genghis Khan, where are the monuments to Alfred Kinsey, Havelock Ellis, Marie Stopes, and Anne de Lenclos? We remember Gatling for inventing the machine gun but forget Fallopio for giving us the condom.

Let us pray, then, for a coming generation of neopagans, that the unsung martyrs of the sex wars may not have suffered in vain. In hopes that the future may be more fun, this study is humbly addressed to those who are content to let the dull debate over sexual permissibilities dribble on as long as it may, who prefer rather to extend their loves to the fullest, and who will declare with Thomas Carew in "A Rapture":

> *Like and enjoy: to will and act is one:*
> *We only sin when love's rites are not done.*

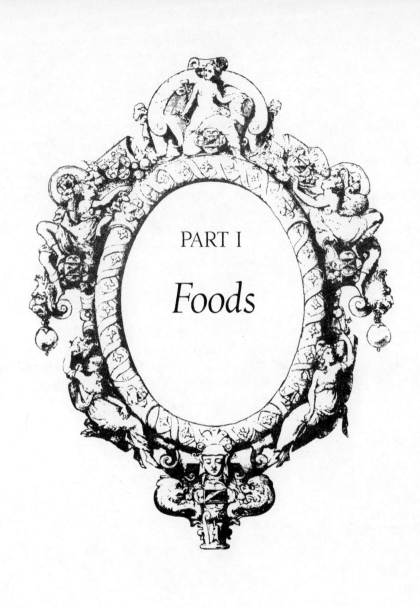

PART I

*Foods*

*Great food is like great sex.*
*The more you have the more you want.*
—GAEL GREENE

*Eat! Drink! Love!*
*For all else is naught.*
—SARDANAPALUS

FROM the first feints and jabs of foreplay to the knockout at the center of the ring, a bout of good loving burns up at least 200 calories in each of the bodies involved—the equivalent of running two miles. If the action is long, intense, or five-in-a-row, the energy outlay can approach that of a marathon.

Overweight women like to make love more often than slender ones, according to psychiatric surveys by Drs. William Shipman and Ronald A. Schwartz in Chicago; similar statistics have been produced at the State University of New York. It's too bad that only women have been subject to the studies, as they already suffer more in the struggle between food propaganda and beauty propaganda. This should not be taken to mean that excess weight is not a health problem or that getting fat will make you horny. But it is absurd that the clotheshorse figure should be the template for all women. Nor does a love of food have to mean fat, let alone the shame in which it is dressed even as our way of life pushes us toward it. The point is that there may be a biological reason why the Cro-Magnons carved those obese figurines of fertility (equals survival; remember it was cold) goddesses. Lust for food and appetite for lust go together like a horse and carriage.

But it seems that many Americans just aren't hungry anymore. There is much talk of the "new chastity," and while it may be mostly talk and no inaction, many people in their twenties and thirties say they've taken themselves off the "market." A decade ago most patients at sex clincs sought help for problems of sexual function, but today about half of them are worried about having no *interest* in sex. Counselors have had to coin a new term: "desire fades." In fact, writers on sex throughout the twentieth century have emphasized a marked decline in the art of love in the industrial nations, as compared with earlier or more "primitive" societies. Is it really only a myth that the good times lasted right up through the eighties and nineties in days of yore?

If not, other reasons are all around us. There are the noise, pollution, overcrowding, and ulcers of our daily hives. There is frustration from constant media titillation. There are widespread inferiority complexes from comparison with sex idols. There is performance anxiety from a too literal interpretation of the sex-sports equation implied at the opening of this section. There is the need to retreat from our recently learned freedom to fuck around, which for many has turned sour without the ability to manage a long, in-depth affair. There is the 1970s malaise of spiritual escapism while impotently watching the world go to hell in a handbasket on television. There is the disillusionment of people who, as one defeatist psychiatrist put it, "expect far too much from their sex lives."

But there's one more reason why we've lost our appetite: our food. Since 1910 our per capita consumption of fresh fruits, vegetables, and whole grains has declined by one-third to three-fourths, depending on the commodity, according to a report of the Center for Science in the Public Interest. The gap has been filled with Ring-Dings, Bloatburgers, Chem-Shakes, and Raspberry-Almond-Ding TV dinners. Is it any wonder we eat and eat but are never satisfied and wither young?

The human body is adaptable; it will survive a surprisingly long time on just about anything. Sexual health, like any other kind of fine health, is more complicated. The first rule is that there are no rules. Each person's nutritional requirements are as individual as a fingerprint. Normal, healthy people have been found to have 10- to 50-fold variations in the efficiency of their enzyme systems; 100- to 200-fold differences in amounts of digestive juices in the stomach; and 3-fold variations in circulatory efficiency. Many persons labeled schizophrenic have been cured once it was realized they had a need for niacin (vitamin $B_3$) up to a thousand times as great as most people's. An average daily requirement for vitamin A has never been set, because individual differences are too great. Experimental nutritionist Dr. Roger Williams has said, "metabolically, the phrase 'average person' has as much meaning as 'average picture.'"

Each of us is faced with the fiendishly difficult task of getting *our best* amounts of forty or fifty essential factors into our bodies every day. Some of these vitamins and minerals are unknown. This has been proven by experiments in which animals have been fed synthetic diets made up of all *known* nutrients. They live, but with each generation they lose vigor and reproductive capacity. The population eventually dies out unless natural foods are added to their diet. The food Americans eat is reflected in subclinical malnutrition in 80 percent of the population, an estimate independently made by several nutritionists, including Dr. Emmanuel Cheraskin and Dr. Carl C. Pfeiffer, based on several national nutritional surveys. The only way to attain optimum nutrition is by a long period of self-education, self-experiment, patience, intelligence, and, if possible, expert guidance.

Fortunately, there are some guidelines which work for almost everybody:

᭞— Look for a happy medium between overeating and undereating. Don't eat unless you're actually hungry, and try not to eat more than you can comfortably digest. Take Norman Douglas's advice: ". . . a fasting stomach and a full one have nothing in common save this: both are enemies to Love."

᭞— Eat it raw. A temperature of 80° C. (176° F.) for just a few minutes is enough to destroy most enzymes found in fresh food. Prolonged cooking destroys vitamin E and many of the B vitamins.

᭞— Preserve your best acid-alkaline balance. Nearly all fresh fruits and vegetables yield a preponderance of alkaline ions in blood and nerves when digested. Most canned, frozen, or dried produce, legumes, flesh foods, grains, nuts (except almonds), and dairy products (except raw milk and yogurt) produce an acid reaction. Since an alkaline-ion reserve is essential for transporting carbon dioxide to the lungs for elimination, more than half of the diet should be alkaline-forming. A 70:30 or 80:20 proportion is usually quoted as ideal. Inefficient $CO_2$ excretion leads to an antisexual fatigue and sluggishness. Acid-forming foods include most of our proteins and nearly all the sexually stimulating foods, so don't try to eliminate them entirely. The nearly identical Chinese and Indian concepts of balancing *yang* or *ragasic* (acid) and *yin* or *sattvic* (alkaline) foods recognized that both are essential.

᭞— The amount and quality of protein should be individually adjusted so as to repair everyday wear and tear and give the organism raw materials for growth—the basis of all tissue-building (anabolic or analeptic) diets. An active sex life increases protein needs for the replacement of hormones as well as the usual restitution after exercise. It does not mean poisoning the body with more protein than it can handle, but rather giving it a bit more than the minimum.

The National Academy of Sciences' Food and Nutrition Board's current estimate is .36 gram per pound of body weight, or 55–60 grams for men and 45–50 grams for women of average build. This includes a generous allowance for individual variation and malabsorption problems, so many people's needs are less. The UN's Food and Agriculture Organization's recommended amounts are about one-third less for all ages, and there is a growing body of evidence that buildup of waste products from digestion of excess protein raises metabolic rate above normal, leading to faster aging. A 150-pound person can get by on only 25 grams of protein daily to replace average metabolic losses, yet most Americans consume close to 100 grams. Unfortunately, the ins and outs of protein selection are too big a topic to tackle here, and I don't know of any one book that does it completely for the nontechnical reader, although Francis Moore Lappé's and Gary Null's are a good start.

❧— Let your body be your guide. This is a risky one, but ultimately, the ability to sense what makes your body feel better or worse is the key to sexual eating. What we now call body wisdom is the same as the doctrine of "enlightened taste" that Brillat-Savarin laid down in *The Physiology of Taste*.

Everyone who makes love believes in aphrodisiacs. Granted, these days the belief is mostly subliminal; many people have never consciously thought about the concept. But we all have at least a favorite dress or perfume, a favorite ascot or aftershave, that helps us get in the groove.

Moreover, the form of the myth reflects those who create it. Those who can't conceive of making love without outside help either feel unsure of their own bodies or see themselves as pawns in cosmic chess. Those who seek aphrodisiacs as a sort of hobby, looking for the odd thrill, see themselves as active participants in a more loosely woven web of existence, where one can to some extent plan one's experiences.

Religious symbolism originally played a large part. Penis- and vulva-shaped pastries baked for fertility deities were eaten by the worshipers for stimulus. Such were the *kamanu* cakes of the Babylonian goddess Ishtar, and though they are less graphic, Chinese New Year moon cakes represent the survival of the same custom, giving thanks for the harvest and praying for next year's fecundity.

Ovid, chary of drugs, states, "The best aphrodisiac is your own passion," but he also recommends honey, pine nuts, eggs, basil, scallions, and rocket. Most other classical writers agree with him, adding only a generous helping of seafood. Horace includes marrow and liver.

While Europeans were either trying to be chaste or relying on medieval magic, the Indians and Arabs were developing their own aphrodisiac cuisines. They found agreement on the virtues of onions and garlic, milk and honey, nuts and legumes, eggs, lamb or mutton, and a huge array of sweet, aromatic, and hot spices.

Jean Liébault, whose sixteenth-century *Treasury of Secret Remedies for the Diseases of Women* actually covers both sexes admirably, heralds the redevelopment of Western amatory cuisine. He speaks warmly of nuts, figs, dates, game, fish with onions, chestnuts, meat cooked so as to be easily digestible, pomegranates, spices, a little wine, and chicken soup—not necessarily in that order.

Liébault's English neighbors had such a large vocabulary of erotic foods, they had to sing little ditties to remember them:

> Good sir if you lack the strength in your back
> And would have a Remediado
> Take Eryngo rootes & Marybone tartes
> Red wine & riche potato.

*An oyster pie & a lobsters thighe*
*hard eggs well dressed in Marow*
*This will ease your backes disease*
*and make you good Cocksparrowe.*

*An Apricock or an Artichock*
*Anchovies oyle and Pepre*
*These to use do not refuse*
*Twill make your backe the better.*

*The milke of an Asse will bringe to Passe*
*all things in such a matter*
*When this is spent you must be contente*
*with an ounce of Synamon water.** 

Dr. Nicolas Venette, author of the mid seventeenth-century *Tableau de l'amour conjugal* (translated by Sir Charles Carrington in 1900 as *Conjugal Love: or the Pleasures of the Marriage Bed Reveal'd*), lauds seminal nutrifiers like egg yolks, cock testicles, crabs, prawns, crayfish, beef marrow, sweet wine, milk, "and such foods as tend to cause wind." France under the two Louises (XIV and XV) combined what survived in Italy of Greek and Roman cooking with the peasants' restorative foods, then added the fruits of exploration—ambergris, chocolate, cloves, et cetera—and elaborated them all into a table not seen since the fall of Rome.

But it was not until the eighteenth century that dining and dallying embraced each other to the fullest. The appearance of distilled liquor aided the growing liberation from churchly strictures, and promiscuity became the upper-class fashion. The brothels' *salles des préparations* became virtual factories of pastilles, herbifications, and elixirs, and they vied with one another for the fortitudination of their tables.

Poor frigid Madame de Pompadour made herself very sick by

* Anonymous broadside

eating nothing but "heating" foods—fish, truffles, mushrooms, asparagus, vanilla, chocolate—while trying to keep up with Louis XV's demands. Madame du Barry's ginger omelets, turtle soup, sweetbreads, shrimp, and celery soup were widely famed for hefting the same scepter. A national tradition of *petits soupers* gained expression in Grimod de la Reynière's remark that ladies are "more amiable at suppertime than at any other hour of the day."

For a simple little supper, a few hors d'oeuvres, a meat or fish dish, a vegetable, a small salad, a light dessert, and but one wine will suffice. The more elaborate dinners follow the "rules" of classic French cuisine—soup, hors d'oeuvres, fish, fowl, meat, vegetable, salad, dessert, liqueur, with wines to match each course.

The ultimate setting for such a meal also evolved under the French monarchy—the *salons particuliers* or *chambres séparées* which survive today in elaborate Parisian restaurants like L'Hôtel and La Pérouse. The doors have no knobs, and plush furnishings center around table and bed, side by side. One aging Lothario, interviewed centuries ago by the Squire of Baudricourt, had even developed a set of menus for blondes, another for brunettes. For golden locks the decor must be blue, scented of heliotrope, with vases of violets and irises. The meal includes lobster, partridge, eggs, peas, and potatoes with a dry Sauterne. Brunettes, he says, glow best amid gold, with verbena and dark roses around a table of sole, eggs, pheasant with a Margaux, asparagus, and a fruit bombe. He suggests a mixture of the two effects for redheads. Now that seduction is a two-way street, go to it, ladies. Let's find out what settings enhance different types of men.

The proper linkage of food and hair color is but one of the unanswered questions of sexual nutrition. We still know few details about how nutrients are turned into hormones, languor, pelvic warmth, and the other tools of the trade. For all we know, some diets may promote the sexual life at the expense of, say, intellect or longevity.

Without waiting for the scientists, our own aphrodisiac research, along with a little honesty, can close the gap between bravado and satisfaction, as voiced in the complaint Shakespeare put in Cressida's mouth, that ". . . all lovers swear more performance than they are able, and yet reserve an ability that they never perform: vowing more than the performance of ten, and discharging less than the tenth part of one."

# Ambergris

ONCE in a great while a grayish black waxy lump floats ashore somewhere along the world's tropical coasts, most often in the Bahamas. With exposure to air and light it gradually gets lighter in color, and its odor changes from faintly fecal to something like oily hyacinths. It is occasionally found in mid ocean. Ancient protophilosophers must have spent years contemplating it, trying to figure out where it came from, which god sent it for what. They rubbed some on their skin; they ate some. The perfume made the menfolk think of Pleistocene panties, and when they ate it, their blood was more amorous.

At some point, when a shore tribe was cutting up a beached sperm-whale carcass, it was found that ambergris comes from the behemoth's bowels. Some pieces contain the undigested beaks of squid, for ambergris is the scab sloughed from the stomach lining when the whale's wounds from the beaks have healed. The lump floats to the surface when the whale belches it up, usually in pieces weighing a few ounces. The known record is 922 pounds.

Naturally, ambergris was often combined with the rest of love's most precious ingredients to rejuvenate rich impotentates. In the heyday of the Persian Empire, pastilles were pressed from powdered gold, pearls, rubies, and the dried whale wax. Myriad recipes followed, and ambergris pills (*avunculae Cypriae*, "aunts of Cyprian Aphrodite") were in much demand in Greece and

Rome. Later, Arab and Turkish rulers liked a cup of coffee poured over a few grains of ambergris. Cardinal Richelieu thought his amber-coated bonbons helped him father a son at eighty-five. According to the scandal sheet "Spy of the Heart," "The attachment of the king [Louis XV] for Madame du Barry came to her through the prodigious exertions she made during an ambered baptism [bath] in which she perfumed herself interiorly every day. One adds that she joined to that a secret which one still does not admit in good company." (In such references *ambre gris* should not be confused with *ambre jaune*—yellow, or Baltic, amber—the fossilized resin of trees. This was also used medicinally, chiefly against asthma, hysteria, the plague, and witchcraft—but has no aphrodisiac history to speak of.)

Aphrodite's aunts sold well in France for centuries after— *tablettes de magnanimité* and *seraglio pastilles*. One of the more elaborate recipes is handed down by the medieval Portuguese doctor Zacutus Lusitanus in his *Praxis Medica Admiranda* ("Admirable Healing Practice"). Unfortunately the amounts of each component must be guessed:

BOLE TUCCINUM—a clod of fine clay, usually tinted with iron oxide, in this case from Tuccinum

MUSK—the dried penile secretion of the musk deer, used in China as a cardiotonic and stimulant in doses of 200–375 milligrams

AMBERGRIS

ALOESWOOD—the resinous wood of the tropical Asian *Aquilaria agallocha*

RED AND YELLOW SANDERS (*Pterocarpus santalinus*)— sandalwood

SWEET FLAG (*Acorus calamus*)

GALANGA—the roots of East Asian *Alpinia officinalis*, like ginger

CINNAMON

RHUBARB

INDIAN MYROBALAN (See Fruit, page 28)

ABSINTHE—wormwood, *Artemisia* genus and "some pounded stones."

Lazare Rivière, in his *First Treatise on Man and His Essential Anatomy*, presents a more exact formula:

AMBER   ½ drachm (30 grains or 1.94 grams)
MUSK   2 scruples (40 grains or 2.59 grams)
ALOES   1½ drachms (90 grains or 5.83 grams)

These are ground together, then covered with a handbreadth of spirits of wine (brandy), distilled slowly by heating a bed of sand in which the flask is embedded, the brew filtered and taken daily in a dose of three to five drops. He hints that it is especially good in a little orange-rose-cinnamon syrup.

Boswell states in his graduate thesis, *Dissertatio Inauguralis de Ambra*, that three grains of ambergris will accelerate the pulse, improve muscular strength and intellectual faculties, and dispose one to cheerfulness and desire. Ambergris is 80 percent cholesterol, a precursor of numerous steroid hormones, so perhaps there is something in it. Chemical analysis shows that it also contains an alcohol called ambrein, benzoic acid, an oil, and $5\beta$–cholestan–$3\alpha$–ol.

Today its major use is in the perfume industry, where a tincture is both a rare fragrance and a fixative for flower scents. It is one of those commodities that literally has no price. A carefully scrutinized buyer-applicant must contract with a supplier for whatever it takes to get the desired amount.

The hunting of sperm whales for ambergris is prohibited by the U.S. Marine Mammal Protection Act. But whales were never really hunted for ambergris, which was much rarer than the ingredients for corset stays or lamplight. French industry spokesmen say that 90 percent of the supply is found on beaches, and only 10 percent in the bellies of industrially killed whales. International Flavors and Fragrances, the major supplier of perfume essences and artificial flavors to industry, no longer provides ambergris, but points out that traces are found in many perfumes. Our chances for trying this one vanish with each sperm whale.

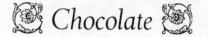 ## Chocolate

ON February 14, 1978, the body of an attractive coed was found on the outskirts of a small New England town. Her clothes were soiled and torn, she could not move, her eyes stared vacantly into space, and she did not even recognize her own family. Her face was covered with ugly brown stains.

The verdict: chocolate.

On April 1, 1978, in Amarillo, Texas, tragedy struck when a mother went berserk and stuffed her three small children into the trash compactor. Neighbors said the toddlers had last been seen running from her, clutching small objects wrapped in tinfoil. A psychiatrist was called in to examine the ominous murky stains found smeared all over the walls of the kitchen and to interpret the woman's disoriented claim that she had been told to do it by a brown devil speaking through the family dog.

The verdict: chocolate.

Day after day reports cross my desk of cases like these, and yet we continue to allow this brown scourge free access to our stores, our homes, and our mouths. Chocolate is our preeminent drug of *direct sexual transference*. I say "drug" advisedly, even though chocolate's nutritional value qualifies it as a food, because its aficionados lust after it as though it were a low-priced brown cocaine. Our streets are filled with men and women wearing puckered, salivaceous smiles, sucking a Swiss egg, a Cadbury, a Hershey's kiss, or a chocolate truffle (that aptly named brown diamond of the gourmet candy shop). But true chocoholics invariably savor their beloved in private, and would resent a sexual encounter with an uncocoa partner as an unpardonable intrusion.

This state of affairs may have something to do with all the rigid bars and sensuously coated Peter Paul Mounds we watched on television during our formative years. Still, advertising cannot explain why hot chocolate has been a special favorite of monks and nuns for centuries. The curious fact remains that chocolate—once considered the most powerful aphrodisiac by American Indians and Europeans, recommended by Havelock Ellis and ballyhooed in the popular advice of nineteenth-century America's Dr. Bushwhacker—has no such reputation today. Instead, it has become a secret *substitute* for love.

Love itself must be getting awfully rare, judging from the three billion pounds of its sepia stand-in consumed yearly—nearly a pound of pure cocoa for every human on the globe. Most of this is eaten in Europe and North America. The Swiss, at twenty-two pounds per person per year, lead the world. Americans, though far behind at a mere ten pounds per person, make up for it in variety with chocolate coins, chocolate soda, chocolate-flavored tobacco and rolling papers, chocolate golf balls, Hershey's "black lightning" syrup straight from the can, and, for the truly lovelorn, Phillips' Chocolate Milk of Magnesia or Chocolated Ex-Lax.

The Mayans must have been almost as desperate, for they drank unsweetened, ground, roasted *cacao* mixed with corn beer, a bitter brew that failed to impress Columbus when he tasted it in 1502 in what is now Honduras. (Our word cocoa, by the way, first appeared in 1755 as an error in Dr. Samuel Johnson's *Dictionary*, and soon supplanted the original spelling.) The Indians of Mesoamerica had been cultivating cocoa for thousands of years, and its status as a nutritious food and sexual stimulant was already well established when the Spaniards came.

Linnaeus followed the Mayans in naming this funny-looking evergreen *Theobroma*, "food of the gods." Its beans were so esteemed that they were used as money throughout the Mayan

Yucatán, even to the point of being hollowed out and filled with dirt by counterfeiters. The Peruvian Indians used cacao as an aphrodisiac and to induce labor in cases of delayed birth; to this day the beans are called *pepe de oro*, "seeds of gold," in Ecuador. Bishop de Landa, Cortes' chaplain, observed that eight to ten beans would buy the "lustful use" of a Mayan public woman.

A thousand miles from the coast, in the Aztec capital of Tenochtitlán, Cortes and his retinue encountered cocoa again, but this time in the form of *xoxo-atl*, a delicious beverage sweetened with honey, flavored with *thilxochitl* (vanilla), and chilled by snow brought by runners from the mountains. Two thousand chalices of this drink were served at court every day, and Montezuma the Last, who was positively addicted, accounted for fifty himself. Although cocoa in some form was apparently drunk by most of the population, Montezuma forbade it to the women of his court. His reasons are unclear; perhaps he merely wanted to increase the potion's reputation by adding the spice of danger, or perhaps he already had enough on his hands, satisfying the demands of his Solomon-sized harem.

Cacao apparently had widespread sexual-religious significance, for large amounts were consumed in the rites of Xochiquetzal, the Aztec goddess of love, akin to Aphrodite. Among the Itzá tribe, it was given to prisoners about to be sacrificed in hopes of turning their hearts to chocolate before offering them to Tonacatecutli, the goddess of food. Cocoa beans also take the place of fire in the Aztec version of the universal myth of Prometheus, known to them as Quetzalcóatl, who was punished by the gods for stealing cocoa beans from the Garden of Life and giving them to man. The prophesied return of this white-skinned cacao-hero from the East was responsible for Cortes' initial reception as a god rather than a plunderer, and so began the downfall of the Indian civilization. Perhaps the wholesale seduction of modern palates by chocolate should be considered Xochiquetzal's revenge for her lost kingdom and sacrifices. (Her tribute was revived in GIs' use of their chocolate bar rations to pay the prostitutes of World War II, Korea, and Vietnam.)

The secret recipe for *xoxo-atl* was gleaned from Montezuma's servants by Cortes' interpreters: Geromino de Aguilar, one of Columbus's sailors shipwrecked on the Yucatán shore and enslaved by the Mayans seventeen years before, and by Donna Marina, an Indian princess also released from Mayan captivity to become Cortes' mistress and translator. During the next several decades chocolate gradually gained immense popularity among the Spanish nobility as cooks learned to modify the Aztec brew to European palates.

In its unsweetened form, cocoa is so bitter that the pirates who preyed on Spanish galleons called it *cacuro de carnero* ("sheep shit") before tossing this part of the cargo overboard. Nevertheless, the fulminations of the clergy against this "provoker of immorality" augmented whatever true aphrodisiac effects it may have and ensured cocoa's popularity among those who could afford it. As late as the seventeenth century, for example, an inquisitor named Marradon accused some ladies of New Spain of learning sorcery from Indian women, who contacted Satan and "committed an infinite number of crimes under the influence of chocolate, of which they were great mistresses." At about the same time, in 1624, Joan Fran Rauch, deploring a current scandal of sexuality among certain monastic orders, said the embarrassment could have been avoided by forbidding the monks this "violent inflamer of the passions."

As irony would have it, it was in a nunnery in Chiapas, Mexico, where sugar, another new discovery, was first added to the beverage around 1550. In the next decade the drink became so popular among the women of the province that they found they could no longer sit through mass without it and had it served to them in church. When the local bishop finally prohibited these indiscretions, most of the parishioners switched to a nearby cathedral, and the good pastor was soon found dead, allegedly from a cup of poisoned chocolate. The conflict was only resolved when Father Escobar, Bishop of Rome, declared a century later that "liquids do not break a fast."

The sweet brew remained a Spanish monopoly until a gentleman named Antonio Carletti brought the recipe to Italy in 1606. Thence it traveled to Austria and thereafter was carried throughout Europe by the female partners of various royal marriages. Anne of Austria brought it to France when she married Louis XIII. But chocolate really became the rage in Paris with the marriage to Louis XIV of the Spanish Infanta, Maria Theresa, whose only two passions were the king and cocoa. The drink was a trusted seduction potion of such famous lovers as Casanova and Madame du Barry.

The bonbons we so casually suck today have resulted from generations of restless experimentation, searching for, in the words of Brillat-Savarin, a chocolate "sweet but not insipid, strong but not bitter, aromatic but not sickly, and thick but free from sediment." The incomparable French gourmet, writing near the end of this exploratory era, describes chocolate mixed with pepper, allspice, aniseed, ginger, musk, orange flowers, rosewater, or the Turkish restorative, salep. The first stage in this process, of course, was the introduction of sugar and vanilla, now integral parts of most chocolates. The modern era dawned with the 1847 invention of solid "eating chocolate," made by adding extra cocoa butter, and the first milk chocolate, made in Vevey, Switzerland, by Daniel Peter and Henri Nestlé in 1876.

The art of making a fine cup of hot chocolate is the same as making a terrible cup of coffee—simmer it gently for ten to fifteen minutes and, if possible, make it a day or two in advance and let it sit at room temperature to give it the slightest tang of fermentation; then reheat. Most recipes tell you to melt bar chocolate in a double boiler so as not to scorch it; this is an excellent start, but if the melted chocolate is then mixed with a little water and carefully cooked over a flame, the result is measurably improved.

Of course, you should start with the finest possible material, an ounce and a half of good semisweet per cup, or perhaps some of the real Mexican chocolate, fragrant with cinnamon and orange peel, available north of the border in chicano groceries or certain urban specialty shops. Extra sugar need not be added to these presweetened types, but even if you use plain old Hershey's cocoa—or better yet, Droste's—the simmering makes a richer cup that needs less than the usual proportion of two parts sugar to one of cocoa.

Hot chocolate should be made in an enamel or porcelain pot to avoid metallic contamination of the taste, and the milk or light cream should be warmed separately, as in café au lait, so it does not curdle while the chocolate is cooking. For an authentic touch, beat the brew till foamy by twirling a wooden spoon in it just as the Mexicans do with their *molinillo*. A pinch of cinnamon, a dash of vanilla or Grand Marnier, a dollop of whipped cream— any of these will add to the effect.

There are almost as many unexcelled chocolate desserts as there are people to swoon over them. This simple classic mousse (from Sylvia Balser Hirsch's delicious *Salute to Chocolate*) is one of the most rewarding nutritional sins ever committed:

*Melt and stir till smooth 8 ounces semisweet chocolate with 3 tablespoons water over hot water in a double boiler. Blend with ½ cup plus 2 tablespoons sweet butter. Separate 6 eggs. Beat 6 yolks till thick, add the chocolate, and beat again, then cool. Whip ½ cup heavy cream, add 5 tablespoons sugar, and whip again. Beat 6 whites till stiff, then fold cream and whites gently into the chocolate. Chill in a glass bowl or mold or 6–8 individual molds.*

The ultimate in aphrodisiac chocolate was, naturally, created by the French. Madame du Barry spiked her king's cups with ambergris, and the good professor, Brillat-Savarin, prescribes a "chocolate of the afflicted," mixed with 72 grains (4.66 grams) of powered ambergris per pound, or a lump the size of a small bean for each cup, for all those who "have drunk too deeply of the cup of pleasure, or given to work too many of the hours which should belong to sleep."

What is there in chocolate that can account for its repute? There is sugar, of course, twanging the sweet tooth and contributing many of the 150 calories in each ounce of bar chocolate, bitter or sweet. There is theobromine, a stimulant very similar to caffeine; it boosts digestive secretions and dilates the bronchioles and the blood vessels of the brain and heart, but stimulates the nervous system less than caffeine. A cup of cocoa has enough (150–200 milligrams) of this alkaloid to produce a recognizable lift, but most eating-chocolate has so little that it is not a factor in any aphrodisiac effect. Several authorities state that wild and early cultivated strains of the cacao tree were much stronger in theobromine, and possibly in nutrients as well.

Chocolate goes through so many stages of preparation—fermenting, drying, roasting, cracking, grinding, pressing to remove cocoa butter, sometimes treatment with an alkali—that it is sometimes assumed that most of its nutritional value is removed by the time it reaches our lips. This is not so. Cocoa is low in vitamins to begin with, but it is rich in minerals, which are not destroyed by the heat of processing. Some physicians used to encourage patients to drink cocoa made from "cracked cocoa" or "cocoa nibs," beans roasted and broken into small pieces without further processing, so as to get the full food value without dilution.

Like all beans, cocoa contains a fair amount of protein, which is not as well balanced in essential amino acids as animal proteins. Only 37 percent of it is usable by the body, but the addition of milk raises this ratio quite a bit. The beans are about 50 percent fat, and cocoa butter is highly saturated, nearly as unhealthful as butter or coconut oil. Cocoa has large amounts of important minerals, including calcium, potassium, and iron, and it is especially rich in phosphorus. As sugar, milk, citric acid, salt, emulsifiers, extra cocoa butter, dyes, and preservatives are added, however, the phosphorus content is substantially lowered. Thus the continuing trend toward eating chocolate rather than drinking it may account in part for its lost reputation as an aphrodisiac.

But to account for its strange metamorphosis from sex drug to sex substitute, we must enter the realm of flavor and texture. The flavor components of the cacao bean stimulate the most sensitive receptors in the mouth—Krause's end-bulbs—to a degree matched by few other foods. Centuries of experimentation with finer grinds and more cocoa butter have created a product that is in a league unto itself as far as "mouth feel" is concerned.

The phosphorus, theobromine, and unique flavor of cocoa are a combination that certainly *could* trigger a sexual reaction, especially among worn-out emperors and love-starved anchorites. But it seems that the reaction of the imbiber predominates over the action of the potion. The early legends of chocolate as a direct and irresistible inflamer may have been a projection by Europeans of their views about "depraved savages" and satanic sex magic onto the reality of a relatively mild stimulant. Today, chocolate's aphrodisiac powers survive in the custom of giving boxed morsels on Valentine's Day, a dim reflection of the Mayan use of these odd brown beans for love or money. It seems we have turned the bitter stimulant into the god of the foods, a placebo as smooth as a woman's breasts. Who is to say which is preferable?

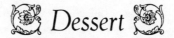 *Dessert*

WHAT more need one say than the last words of Pierette, Brillat-Savarin's sister, shortly before her hundredth birthday: "Bring on the dessert . . . I think I am about to die."

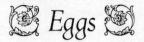

# Eggs

THE egg—one of the shortest nouns in English. We had to give it an extra *g* just to lend it a little weight. The egg—primeval source of us all, the beginning of everything in our individual experience, the almost self-sufficient capsule of new life. The human egg matures in the ovary, a life factory of such roiling ferment that medical illustrations of it look like van Gogh's *Starry Night*. She (for an egg is female until fertilized) ruptures through the ovary wall and sets out on her journey several millimeters long into one of the Fallopian tubes. Her plunge recalls our first cellular lessons of fear and wonder. True, there is the fringed (fimbriated) Fallopian entrance waving her in, bending to follow her course, and perhaps using chemical attraction to reel her in. Floating in the peritoneal sea, perhaps she little dreams of the horde of squiggly pinpoints who long for her massive yolk, rising like the sun at the end of an even longer dark journey.

No wonder many early mythologies say the creation of the universe began with the hatching of a cosmic egg. How could a food so life-central in its essence not be so in its assimilation? The egg's aphrodisiac signature is written all over her. People have always read it so, judging from the unanimity of folklore on this point (some Iranian brides still break eggs on the floor so that the hymen may break as easily), and from the nearly 300 billion eggs eaten every year throughout the world.

Birds have always been considered especially sexy, from the twittering sparrows that drew Aphrodite's chariot to the fierce hawk that personified Eros, and it is their eggs that are most often eaten, although the Egyptians once had a fondness for lizard eggs and the Mayans transmitted their taste for turtle eggs to the French by way of Spain. Many Chinese credit their preserved eggs with more potency than fresh ones. The Romans loved ova so much that an offer to "cook eggs" was a standard come-on, so when champion banqueter Athenaeus quotes cookbook author Heraclides as saying peacock eggs are sweetest, the conclusion rests on considerable research. Modern-day chef Raymond Oliver, who rates plover and pewit (lapwing) as the best, praises the fortifying virtues of duck eggs—raw, scrambled with truffles, or thus deviled with avocado:

*Gently boil 6 duck eggs 12 minutes in lightly salted water to cover. Chill in cold water. Peel and carefully remove yolks, leaving whites as halves. Peel and dice half a ripe avocado. Sieve the other half with 1 tsp. curry powder, 3 pinches celery salt, and a dessert spoon of coconut milk. Mix with mashed egg yolks, fill whites, and garnish with diced avocado.*

Hen's, of course, are the eggs we usually mean in today's kitchen, and the quintessence of fowl appears at the center of most nations' aphrodisiac folklore. Millions of men have gulped a raw egg yolk in their brandy "to put lead in the pencil"—even with no one to write to—ever since the Renaissance, whence comes this strengthening posset, passed on in Norman Douglas's *Venus in the Kitchen:*

### GINESTRATA
*Beat 6 large egg yolks, slowly adding 1 glass Madeira, 1 cup cold chicken broth, and 1 teaspoon ground cinnamon. Smooth texture by passing through a sieve or beating briefly. Cook gently in an earthen pot, stirring constantly, and adding a small pat of butter. As it thickens, pour into cups and serve hot with a sprinkling of nutmeg and sugar.*

For centuries, English parsons gave newlyweds sack possets like this while blessing them at bedside just before the first round of connubial bliss.

There are many variations on the flip, as all egg and alcohol combinations are called. Here is one of the most interesting:

> In a Madeira glass pour ¼ glass Maraschino. Add 1 egg yolk (don't break it). Add ¼ glass mixed Madeira and crème de cacao. Add ¼ glass brandy. Serve without mixing and drink in one gulp.

Casanova often recommended himself to a lady's bed by assuring her that "I have taken nothing today but a cup of chocolate and a salad of eggs dressed with oil from Lucca and Marseilles vinegar. . . . I shall be all right when I have distilled the whites of the eggs, one by one, into your amorous soul."

Among all champions of the egg, however, the Shaykh Nefzawi stands in a class by himself. His discussion of eggs is saved for the last and most important chapter of *The Perfumed Garden for the Soul's Delectation*. In it the wily old shaykh tells his longest tale, "The History of Zohra," whose heroine sets up prodigious tests of cockery for Abou el-Heidja and his two cavalier companions before she will grant el-Heidja her favors. Mimoun, the black, must swive Zohra's friend Mouna as often as she likes for fifty days without tiring. For food he asks only for ample raw egg yolks and bread, then enjoys his task so much he adds an extra ten days just for fun.

What better parable to drive home the moral: Suck eggs. The chieftain's primary aphrodisiac recommendation is the deglutition (swallowing) of raw egg yolks every day, first thing in the morning, before any other food is taken. He also praises eggs boiled with myrrh, cinnamon, and pepper. If one is beset with opportunity before having begun this regimen, he suggests a last-minute booster of scrambled eggs with honey.

There is good reason to take Nefzawi's advice. An average-sized egg provides about 6.75 grams of the highest quality protein. Its essential amino acids—the ones our bodies can't synthesize—are in the proper proportions for human tissue to use almost all of them in building proteins. Some nutritionists believe that milk protein can equal eggs in biological value, but no food except bee pollen surpasses them.

Eggs also contain significant amounts of most vitamins except vitamin C. They are rich in vitamin A, supply some vitamin E and B vitamins (notably pantothenic acid), and are one of the few foods that contain vitamin D. Eggs provide large amounts of minerals, including calcium, iron, potassium, and sodium; they are especially rich in phosphorus. The yolks provide lecithin. Their shells protect them from invading bacteria and from the kind of chemical tampering man has done to most other foods. The shells provide extra calcium and trace minerals—if one eats eggs crunchy whole as our ancestors did or blenderized as advised by some whole-food advocates.

Most of the nutrients and the best protein are concentrated in the nucleus, or yolk. Large eggs, with their disproportionately larger yolks, can be up to one and a half times as nutritious as an equal weight of small ones. Whenever possible, one should eat the yolk and white separately. The yolk is at its best raw—its stock of enzymes and easily digested proteins is damaged by heat. The white is better cooked; raw, one of its enzymes, avidin, binds itself to biotin, one of the B vitamins, and prevents the body from absorbing it. The irony is that biotin, essential to form many of the enzymes used to assimilate fatty acids and amino acids, is abundant in the yolks. Thus the egg, unless separated, begs to be coddled.

The egg is the center of a nutritional controversy between the advocates of high-priced organic foods and the cheaper mass-produced variety. One side claims that only eggs laid by chickens that have been allowed to run free and supplement their grain diet with worms, bugs, grass, and seeds can reach their full nutritional potential. They say that fertilized eggs provide nutritional factors that unfertilized ones do not, and that the same reasoning applies to the meat of the bird herself.

The other side responds that all eggs are the same as long as the hen is fed a balanced diet, and that it is easier for her to get all the nutrients she needs from a commercial mash. The fact that she never moves and sees neither daylight nor rooster does not affect the egg, they explain, nor are antibiotic and preservative residues from the feed significant for human consumers.

The argument between organicists and syntheticists is reminiscent of old theological disputes between materialists and spiritualists, nominalists and realists. Neither side will ever convince the other, because they have no premises they can agree on.

Egg-factory advocates point out that the color of the yolk does not reflect nutritional value, but only the content of xanthophylls, pigments that organic hens pick up from the grasses they eat. For my part, though, ever since I first tasted the thick, dark-orange, nut-flavored yolks of buck-fifty organic jumbos, I have been unable to enjoy the often watery, lemon-colored broth at the center of supermarket eggs. It's hard enough to make do with hen's eggs at all after sampling fresh duck eggs or the enormous, meaty golden feast laid by the goose.

One other egg dispute *has* been unscrambled in the past few years. People with high blood-cholesterol levels were once told to eliminate eggs from their diets to decrease the risk of heart attacks. It has since been learned that this advice did not take into account several important facets of the complex cholesterol problem.

First of all, cholesterol is an essential nutrient; if the body does not get it from food, our tissues will synthesize their own, perhaps in abnormally large amounts. Second, atherosclerotic deposits on artery walls are not caused by high levels of cholesterol circulating in the blood, but rather by deficiencies of one or more nutrients needed for its utilization. Most of these substances are found in egg yolks; one, lecithin, is especially plentiful. Experimental nutritionist Carl Pfeiffer surmises that high energy levels are correlated with an individual's ability to maintain a fairly large amount of cholesterol in the blood because of a nutrient-rich diet that includes two or three eggs a day.

These conclusions have been documented by a great deal of research. One of the most interesting studies involved ten young men who were asked to eat three eggs a day. Some showed only a minuscule rise in serum cholesterol (2 milligrams percent), while others showed a much larger average increase of 27 milligrams percent. The latter group were all smokers and thus inhaled daily doses of poisonous cadmium, a metal that blocks adsorption of the zinc in eggs that would otherwise have enabled their bodies to maintain normal amounts of circulating cholesterol.

In short, as long as you can kick or avoid the smoking habit, you may feel free to enjoy (if you can afford) such classics as Madame du Barry's recipe for deviled plover eggs:

*Stuff a dozen hard-boiled, halved plover eggs with a mixture of their yolks, truffles, and pâté de foie gras. Place them in a casserole lined with bacon to keep them from sticking to the bottom; add some Madeira, a bunch of assorted herbs, a little gravy, and season with salt, pepper, and nutmeg. Then take cooked artichoke bottoms, form them into a cup by pressing in the centers, and fill them with a minced poultry stuffing. Sprinkle them with consommé and place them in the casserole as well. Cover and poach in the oven. Arrange the eggs and artichokes on a platter along with some sautéed rooster kidneys, and ladle over all some game concentrate and a bit of sauce glacé.*

# 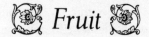 Fruit

*She's a plum.*
*You're peachy.*
*I want your cherry.*
*Give him the fig.*
*You're the apple of my eye.*
*What a pair of melons.*

FRUITS are the leading symbols in humanity's edible complex. Since these succulent epithets are more often applied to women than to men, some feel they encourage males to think of females as mere produce, worthless if too green or overripe; but such an attitude is created by arrogance or fear, not by metaphor. On the whole, these figures of speech do us no harm and add a certain juice to the language. What associations could be more natural when a strawberry is exploding on the tongue or the juice of an exquisite persimmon is dripping down the chin?

What does fruit offer the lover besides the power of suggestion? Sugar. Sweetness is the taste that is closest to our pleasure centers, probably because sugar is the primary fuel of every cell in our bodies and the *only* fuel our brain can burn. Salt has occasionally been considered sexy—hence an occasional "salty" story and the term "salty dog," meaning originally a bitch in heat, but now, perhaps via the image of a hot dog, also meaning the taste of a penis. Sour and bitter are the antithesis of sex to our brain's taste receptors. Sugar is the gastronomic equivalent of sex to every tongue in the world.

That's *almost* the whole story. Fresh fruit supplies some potassium (the most widely distributed of all nutrients) and other minerals. Peaches, mangoes, and Shakespeare's beloved "apricocks" are fairly rich in vitamin A. Many others supply vitamin C, and, when fresh, all are refreshing ways to keep the blood at its proper, slightly alkaline, pH. But there are only a few fruits that figure *as foods* in the legends of aphrodisia, and even fewer that do so for any discernible reason.

The amazing taste and juiciness of the pineapple, mango, and papaya are sufficient reason for their reputation as love fruits, but they also supply vitamins A and C. In addition, papaya contains the enzyme papain, which aids in protein digestion and is used as a meat tenderizer; pineapple supplies the similar enzyme, bromelin.

The ancient Syrian-Hebrew wedding choruses rewritten around 300 B.C. as the Song of Solomon have immortalized the pomegranate in the red of the bride's cheeks. The *Kama Sutra* suggests pomegranate seeds for enlarging the penis; Pliny the Elder hails the pith of the shrublike tree as an aphrodisiac. Neither claim has much support. Pomegranate is rich in vitamin C but contributes little else to the bed table besides its ruby cells.

If symbolism were the measure of aphrodisia, this book would be mostly about apples. To the ancient Greeks and Romans they were love tokens in the same way frat pins, class rings, and chocolates are to us. Many cultures have had a Garden of Eden myth, and in most of them the apple or its local equivalent has been the symbol of erotic joy or sin, depending on the religion's sexual outlook.

The Biblical "apple" (first so identified by St. Jerome in the 4th century A.D.) was probably a quince; pre-Christian apples grew wild by the Black Sea and in Macedonia but were found in only a few other parts of Europe and the Middle East. Throughout this area the quince was one of the most important symbols of the White Goddess, prehistoric mother of the world from whose erotic aspect Aphrodite later developed, who kept the fragrant quince trees blooming in the temples. Like apples, quinces hold only small amounts of several common nutrients, but when baked

(45 minutes to 1 hour at 350° F.) they yield such a buoyantly perfumed sweetness that there just might be something more than symbolism there after all.

From Southeast Asia comes *Phyllanthus emblica,* also known as emblic, myrobalan, or *anvallí*. An inch or two long and very sour, it was recommended to the amorous by Avicenna and most of the Hindu love manuals. The emblic owes its minor reputation to vitamin C, as does the West Indian or Barbados cherry (*Malpighia* genus), which packs an astonishing 1.8 grams per 3 ounces.

The banana has often been proclaimed an aphrodisiac by its shape. Moreover, since it, the date, and the avocado are less watery and more filling than most fruits, all three have been suggested as fortifying foods. (The Aztecs, who called avocados "testicles," made their virgin girls stay home during the avocado season.) But their only stimulant is natural sugar. Claims that these three foods are useful sources of protein are in error, for they all have less than watercress. Nor is there reason to believe that the fruit of the mastic tree (*Pistacia lentiscus*) really builds "strength for coitus," as asserted in *The Perfumed Garden.*

Today there remains only one exotic fruit whose sexual fame cannot be shown to be mostly a product of the mind.

Every August, from all parts of Asia, people journey to Thailand, Indonesia, Malaysia, and the Philippines for the durian harvest, because, as an old Malay proverb tells it, "When the durians fall, the sarongs rise." So provocative is this fruit that the late Indonesian president Sukarno kept a discreet house near Bangkok for feasts and love bouts in the durian season. It is so highly prized that one tree can be its owner's livelihood, and an orchard means great wealth.

*Durio zibethinus* is a huge tree, up to one hundred feet tall, resembling an elm; it usually grows dispersed among other species, although there are still forests entirely of durian in the wilds of Sumatra and Malaysia.

Always wear a pith helmet when strolling under the durians.

*Duri* is Malay for "thorn," and the heavy, football-sized fruits are covered with husks of tough, pyramidal spines that can disable the unwary as they plummet ripe to the ground. They are gathered as soon as they fall by the owner or his watchman, who sits day and night in a nearby hut to grab the bounty as soon as it hits the ground and guards it from human and animal poachers. Next morning the durians go to the local market; they can only be sold locally because they ferment and become inedible within a few days.

Much has been written of the durian's aroma, summed up by one gourmet's famous appraisal: "To say it smells like rotten garlicky cheese is generous." The early Dutch colonists banned *doeren* or *duryoen* from their settlements, and even today some Southeast Asian airlines and hotels refuse to serve it. Every autumn the English-language paper in Kuala Lumpur prints a feature on Western noses' reactions. Oddly enough, most Asian aficionados find the odor less objectionable than a German does Limburger cheese. The clue may lie in the Malay claim that alcohol and durian are a dangerous, even lethal, combination. Teetotaling Westerners who enjoy even the smell have reported that those who most hate it also seem to drink the most.

All who try it agree on the flavor of the rich custardy pulp. First described to the English-speaking world by Victorian naturalist A. R. Wallace as a buttery almond with hints of onion, sherry, and cream cheese, the taste and texture bring immediate sexual associations. Scooping out the lush flesh with the tongue is perhaps the closest one can get to cunnilingus without a woman.

As far as I know, durian has not been chemically analyzed, but the Chinese consider it so full of protein they advise pregnant women to eat sparingly of it for fear of bearing a child too big for the birth canal. In any case, durian's effect seems to go far beyond mere power of suggestion. Soon after eating, a warm glow of relaxed animal excitement invades the body, leading to erections, erotic reveries, and/or sensuous love, depending on the circumstances. Durian sellers get more on-the-job propositions than any other occupational group except prostitutes. Don't be a glutton, though. An acquaintance once described a durian overdose: After his third in one morning, the sexual arousal gave way to high fever and profuse sweat. After an hour's discomfort, he was left with a feeling of light-headedness that lasted till the next day. Van Linschoten, in his 1596 account of a voyage to the East, reported that one or two betel leaves will quickly cure the fever. Despite the results of overindulgence, a Malay proverb says, "A man can never have enough durian."

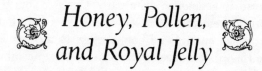

# Honey, Pollen, and Royal Jelly

> Then, as the empty Bee, that lately bore
> Into the common treasure all her store,
> Flies 'bout the painted field with nimble wing,
> Deflow'ring the fresh virgins of the Spring—
> So will I rifle all the sweets that dwell
> In thy delicious paradise, and swell
> My bag with honey, drawn forth by the power
> Of fervent kisses from each spicy flower.
> —THOMAS CAREW, from "A Rapture"

HONEY is nature's metaphor for sex, the stickum that holds all the species together, just as the amber glue itself binds the ingredients of Chinese aphrodisiac pills. Viscous lake on the reveling tongue, a spoonful of honey, after helping the medicine go down, dissolves into bliss like no other eat-treat. Love's first month is its honey-moon. Honeyed water was a favored medium to float lovers close to each other in the *balnea mixta* of Greek and Roman public baths, the inner chamber where all good aristocrats came, to each other's aid, more than two thousand years before the opening of Plato's Retreat. The oldest known love song is an epithalamium sung in the twenty-first century B.C. by the queen to her new husband, Sumerian King Shu-Sin:

> Bridegroom, dear to my heart,
> Goodly is your beauty, honeysweet,
> Lion, dear to my heart,
> Goodly is your beauty, honeysweet.

No one knows when humanity grew its first sweet tooth, although there is evidence that ancient peoples used honey mainly as a medicine, a base for mead (see Alcohol, page 156), and a ceremonial food—in rites that we can now only fondly imagine. Even though they had efficient hive systems—which in Egypt were floated up and down the Nile on barges to follow the ripening blossoms—our ancestors came nowhere near our own sugar consumption. This is just as well, for honey is so refined that an excess of it can be almost as damaging as our average hundred pounds of sucrose per person every year. Nevertheless, the golden elixir does have several useful ingredients that Domino doesn't.

The sweet, watery flower nectar is digested in the bees' stomachs, then thickened as they let it drip slowly down their protruding proboscises to evaporate most of the water in the hot, dry hive. Most of the plants' sucrose, a disaccharide, is broken down into more easily digested monosaccharides—levulose (also called fructose, or fruit sugar, an essential component of semen) and dextrose (or glucose). These mirror-image molecules are honey's main ingredients, usually in the ratio of 40 percent levulose to 30 percent dextrose.

There is no truth to the myth that honey is safe for diabetics and hypoglycemics. Yet because fructose is converted to glucose and burned for energy without stimulating insulin flow, honey is about 40 percent less harmful to them than table sugar.

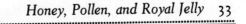
*Honey, Pollen, and Royal Jelly* 33

For the rest of us honey is the safest, fastest, most easily absorbed energy food. Iron pumpers lick it between sets. Other athletes use it for extra oomph before the race or game and for quick recovery afterward. Sir Edmund Hillary took it to the peak of Everest, and several scientific experiments have confirmed its place as number-one sports pickup.

Boudoir gymnasts have long known honey's powers in the amatory olympics, even if they didn't know that easily absorbed sugar is essential for quick replenishment of semen. The Moroccans recognize this fact when they begin their wedding celebrations, sometimes called orgies, with a feast of honey cakes and honey ales. So did the ancient Egyptian bridegrooms, who had to promise as part of the marriage vow to give their mates twenty-four hins (thirty-two pounds) of honey.

Honey is perhaps the easiest of all aphrodisiacs to use. You don't even need a spoon. In fact, finger-lickin' can lead to all sorts of other ideas. Just don't forget to change those expensive satin sheets before you spread it all over each other. (By the way, it's a wonderful *anti*lubricant if you find you need a little more friction in the vagina.)

Many aphrodisiac recipes with other main ingredients use honey to add to the effect. For example, the Shaykh Nefzawi recommends a precoital snack of twenty almonds and one hundred pine nuts with a small glass of honey. The good shaykh also recommends an ambrosia of camel's milk and honey to keep the virile member "always on the alert."

Every culture has its favorite recipe for honey cake or honey bread, from the *medivnyk* of the Ukraine to France's marvelous *pain d'épices*. But for a quick and easy prelude to amour, few dishes can beat the following Chinese apple salad:

> Core and thinly slice 2 large apples. Blend a dressing from the juice of 1 orange, 4 teaspoons of honey, or more to thicken it, and a dash of brandy. Garnish with raisins, walnuts, and fresh cherries. Serves 2.

Although it is primarily levulose and dextrose with smaller amounts of thirteen other sugars, honey also includes traces of other substances. Flavor is imparted by a taste bud's kaleidoscope of alcohols, esters, terpenes, and aldehydes that combine to make as many honey vintages as there are wines. The organic acids include aspartic, one of the nonessential amino acids. According to still inconclusive medical research, an increased supply of aspartic acid may improve stamina, and some doctors have used it to treat "bedroom fatigue" in women.

Honey is well tolerated by the body because it contains many vitamins and minerals needed for sugar metabolism: thiamine ($B_1$), riboflavin ($B_2$), niacin ($B_3$), pyridoxine ($B_6$), biotin, pantothenic acid, potassium, sulfur, calcium, sodium, phosphorus, magnesium, silicon, iron, manganese, and copper. Honey aids in the adsorption of calcium from other dietary sources and improves the hemoglobin count of the blood. But only raw, unheated honey has the full complement of nutrients, for many are lost in the heating and filtering of the supermarket variety. Dark honeys contain up to ten times as much of them as the light ones. And beware of labels, even in health-food stores. Business-oriented Food and Drug Administration regulations allow honey producers to label as "uncooked" those that have been heated to 160° F. so it flows easily enough for machine bottling. From a nutritional standpoint, such honey is no longer as the bees made it; look instead for the word "unheated."

All that processing is unnecessary for shelf life, because honey contains a bactericide called inhibin, making it one of the few natural foods that can be stored without refrigeration, although it will eventually ferment if the air is moist. Honey has kept in perfect condition for three or four thousand years in arid Egyptian graves. Because of its germicidal action and water attraction, honey can even make people more lovable by healing sores, burns, rashes, slashes, and inflamed skin.

Distilled sunlight can be used straight from the comb or jar for many skin irritations, but the classic recipe is this facial.

> Combine ⅓ cup finely ground oatmeal with about 3 teaspoons honey and 1 teaspoon rosewater. Relax under the face pack for half an hour, wash it off with warm water, then rinse with cold water or an astringent. Continued applications once a week usually improve pimply or oily skin.

Then there's Queen Anne's hair lotion (for brunettes only), revealed by her hairdresser only after her death:

> Mix 2 parts honey to 1 part olive oil, massage into the hair near a warm fireplace or its equivalent for 20 minutes, then shampoo.

Anne Stuart credited her four to eight treatments per year with keeping her tresses lustrous long after youth had flown.

There's also evidence that honey helps keep that sweet bird around longer, while preserving vitality for bed-play. When Soviet biologist Nikolai Tsitsin sent a research questionnaire to Russian centenarians, he found a surprising percentage of them were beekeepers. This is the same result reached almost two thousand years ago in a survey described by Pliny the Elder in his *Natural History.* Pliny found a hotbed of longevity in honey-rich northern Italy and on the "Honey Isle of Beli," as Britain was then known. Further classical recommendations came from Galen and Ovid in Rome and Pythagoras, Hippocrates, Apollonius, and Democritus in Greece, where there are still more hives per square mile than anywhere else in the world. All lived a long and sensual life that they credited, at least in part, to a daily ration of the gold of the gods. For their ambrosia, the ancients, mortal and immortal, prized above all others the wild thyme nectar from Mount Hymettus near Athens.

Beekeepers may owe their long lives to business integrity, for they sell the clear amber to their customers and keep the "dirty residue" for themselves. The leftovers are almost pure pollen, one of the most intriguing foods in nature. Before there were beekeepers there were thieves, and the price of larceny in this case is eternal stings. One of humankind's first works of art shows the price of honey so high it may not have been worth it unless for something even more precious. At Cuevas de Araña (Spider's Caves) in Spain about 13,000 B.C., near the end of Old Stone Age culture, a hunter climbs a cliff face on a primitive ladder, probably made of grass, one hand holding and filling a basket with combs while the other wields a smoky torch against the angry swarm, enormously enlarged.

The reward was a raw feast of pollen, bee grubs, royal jelly—if the queen were taken—the wax comb and, oh yes, sweet balm for those pulsating stings. Beebread, beevert, or bee pollen, rich in protein, is one of nature's most complete foods, containing all twenty-two of the elements known to compose the human body. As flower sperm, it is seminal to bees as well, being the one essential food they need to grow from larvae into adults. Drones, the shiftless males who live on welfare all their lives just to train for their shot at pricking the queen, must have lots of pollen to develop sperm, and they are fed it, predigested, by the worker-females.

A bee can gather four million pollen grains an hour. She moistens them with some of the nectar digesting in her stomach, then sticks them together in two 10-milligram pellets carried in the baskets of hair on her hind legs. After all that work she is then robbed by the pollen trap invented by French beekeepers—a screen with openings small enough to dislodge the pellets as the bee struggles through to the hive.

The thousand or so pellets in a teaspoon, the most often recommended daily dose, pack an astounding concentration of nutrients. Pollen averages higher in protein than meat, eggs, or cheese, but its percentage of essential amino acids is three to four times that of any other food. The vitamin B content can be one quarter of total weight. For example, University of Minnesota botanists in the 1940s found these vitamin levels in *one gram* of bee pollen:

| | |
|---|---|
| thiamine ($B_1$) | 9.2 mg. |
| riboflavin ($B_2$) | 18.5 |
| niacin ($B_3$) | 200. |
| pyridoxine ($B_6$) | 5. |
| pantothenic acid | 30–50. |

Pollen also contains appreciable amounts of vitamins A, C, and E, as well as the minerals potassium, magnesium, calcium, phosphorus, sulfur, manganese, iron, and copper. Other components are 10–15 percent sugars, a rainbow of pigments from white through yellow and red to green and black, enzymes and hormones, and an antibiotic. Pollen also contains rutin, a nutrient that has been shown to strengthen capillary walls and add power to the contractions of the heart while slowing its rhythm.

The gonadotropic (sex-organ-stimulating) hormones of most plants are similar to human gonadotropin secreted by the pituitary. And one kind of pollen, from the date palm, contains exactly the same hormone molecule, confirming the ancient Bedouin use of this medicine for sterility. Doctors in Sweden, led by Dr. Ask-Upmark of Uppsala and others from the University of Lund, have found a pollen extract called cernilton very effective in treating prostatitis, and now it is being used in the United States.

There is, however, a controversy as to how much bee pollen humans can use. Pollen grains have tough walls that fossilize so well they are one of our best ways of knowing what plants grew in bygone eons. Some pollen can resist acids as strong as aqua regia, so there is doubt about how much is digested. We don't know the dose favored by the ancient Egyptians, Chinese, Greeks, or Persians, but some modern proponents warn against more than a teaspoon a day, believing that more acts as a stimulant. In munching up to three or four tablespoons a day for several weeks, I have found this warning unfounded. After a teaspoon or so, I noted the faint but pleasantly definite stimulus of a concentrated food, but a larger intake did not seem to produce correspondingly greater results.

Another consideration is that pollen can be heavily laced with pesticides if it comes from flowers near sprayed farmland. Unfortunately, there is no way around this problem except by personally investigating your source. This may not be a major problem for humans, though, because bees that visit sprayed flowers often die before they get back to the hive. But a diabolical new insecticide—microscopic Penncap-M parathion pellets, the same size as pollen grains—may soon pose a threat to the entire bee population as well as to humans who eat honey and pollen.

The heart of the bee colony is the hive, the heart of the hive is the queen, and her heart won't beat without royal jelly. A small amount is fed to all larvae just before they emerge as adults, but an abundance of it is required by the queen throughout her life. The royal virgin who first chews her way out of her egg cell stings all her unemerged rivals to death. Later, a ten- to thirty-minute nuptial flight is her one brief encounter with love as, pursued by a comet's tail of horny drones, she leads the pack until the one who scores fills her with enough sperm to last her lifetime; then the drone often falls dead to earth with his penis broken off like Cochise's arrow in her vagina. Royal jelly is virtually the queen's only food just before this escapade and throughout the egg-laying years that follow.

A concentrate secreted by the workers during pollen digestion, the jelly is thin and milky, two-thirds protein, loaded with B complex, C and D vitamins, and protected by the antibiotic 10–hydroxy–decanoic acid. Royal jelly is the richest natural source of pantothenic acid, and even includes an enzyme that raises adsorption of this vitamin above normal human limits. In animal experiments, pantothenic acid has added 19 percent to the life-span of mice, increased their litter size, and improved hatchability of hen's eggs. Its effects on reproduction are untested in humans. Because of pantothenic acid's importance to the adrenal glands in their production of cortisone, royal jelly has been found beneficial to rheumatoid arthritics. But so far there seems to be no reason to think it is a wonder food for the general populace. One problem is the price. Even for a queen bee, it's sometimes hard to get enough. For all who wish to experiment, however, fresh jelly in capsules is preferable to the desiccated powder form.

> *He saw, in a far valley, a separate grove*
> *Where the woods stir and rustle, and a river,*
> *The Lethe, gliding past the peaceful places,*
> *And tribes of people thronging, hovering over,*
> *Innumerable as the bees in summer*
> *Working the bright-hued flowers, and the shining*
> *Of the white lilies, murmuring and humming.*
> —VERGIL, from *The Aeneid,* Book VI

Thus Aeneas sees a vision of one of the oldest symbolisms, that which represents the soul as a bee. Throughout human history, honey has oozed through some of our strongest religious and sexual beliefs. The Egyptians fed honey to their sacred animals and dipped corpses in it as part of the embalming process. All three of the Aryan Hindu gods—Vishnu, Krishna, and Indra—are Madhava, "nectar-born"; Vishnu is further depicted as a bee on a lotus, while Krishna, Vishnu's earthly incarnation, is often shown as a bee on Vishnu's forehead. Bengalese Brahmans still anoint the bride's head, lips, eyelids, and earlobes with honey at the wedding—so the gods might reside in her and make her divinely sweet.

Several ancient tribes of the Far East spread honey on the bride's breasts and vulva in the name of fertility—to attract the bee-souls. Modern lovers follow a hallowed tradition when they spread their partners with bee candy. Truly, as Victor Hugo crystallized it, "Life is a flower of which love is the honey." But perhaps the best is yet to come—in the 3.75 percent of honey that is still unanalyzed, listed as "undetermined matter" in the chemical breakdowns. That may be the bee's knees.

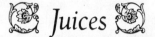 Juices

JIZZUM is the flower of a man's blood. It takes about forty hours to restore its supply fully after an ejaculation. One of the goals of aphrodisiac eating is to lessen this time as much as possible, for the sensation of fullness adds much to the male's readiness, willingness, and ability.

Semen is a joint product, a mix of secretions from several organs. While the sperm cells, born in the testes, are maturing in the epididymis, they are bathed in a fluid rich in potassium, sodium, and glyceryl-phosphoryl-choline. The last is an energy source for sperm motility. While stored in the ampulla or urethral bulb, they swim in the prostatic fluid, loaded with zinc and with proteolysins and fibrolysins to clear a path for the sperm. Just before their daddy comes and they go, they are doused with the largest part of the fluid they swim in—from the seminal vesicles. This provides vitamin C, more citric acid, phosphorus, a reducing (oxygen-removing) compound called ergothioneine, the hormones prostaglandin, vesiglandin, adrenaline, and noradrenaline, and a large supply of fructose for the wigglers to eat.

It all adds up to 95 percent protein and only 2 calories. It's really concentrated. Why, did you know that once, years ago, a crew of whalers were in the habit of whacking off into a tub of sperm oil? Candles were eventually made from that consignment of oil and a conventful of nuns got immaculately pregnant. (Gershon Legman traces this combination gospel parody and potency joke to mid-1920s Scranton, Pennsylvania.)

The Kukukuku headhunters of New Guinea make semen's compact power the center of adolescent male education. Their culture programs exclusive homosexuality for teenagers, and no boy can grow to manhood and marriage, they say, without a steady diet of male essence. Their equally ferocious neighbors, the Marind-Anim, hold a ceremony called the *otiv-bombari*. Each young woman, before her wedding night and after recovering from the birth of each child, must fuck every man in her husband's clan one after the other. The semen that drips out is collected in coconut shells to be used in medicinal foods and ointments. The Marind-Anim women, although they don't enjoy the rite, consider it a sure cure for infertility.

Semen's magical power to distill a child from a few drops of jelly has been one of the male's chief justifications of supremacy. Before the discovery of human eggs in the nineteenth century, men often claimed women were mere baby jars for life, which came wholly from come. However, though not so copious, proteinaceous, or well studied, vaginal secretions are vivifying in their own right. They include acid mucus, perfumes, lubricant "sweated" directly from the blood through the vaginal wall, and other juices from several small glands whose precise function is not yet known. For some strange evolutionary reason, the blood, hormones, and uterine lining of the menses are not reabsorbed by women as they are by other primate females. Perhaps nature meant us to use the fluid as an aphrodisiac—and we have, usually as a secret ingredient in bread (see page 210).

Nor should we neglect the spiritual nourishment derived from approaching near enough to taste the gate of the womb. Dining at the Y is probably as close to Eden as we can expect to get, but for the woman's nutritional counterpart of semen, please turn to Milk, page 55.

# 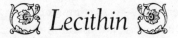 Lecithin

GREAT things have been promised to consumers of a dietary supplement called lecithin. As far back as the Gay Nineties it was promoted in reducing aids as "the fuel that burns body fats," and today these claims have been broadened to include amelioration of diabetes, lowering of intraocular pressure in glaucoma, prevention or treatment of fatty liver, protection against cholesterol deposits on artery walls, and even as a cure for the heartbreak of psoriasis. The surprising thing is that most of these claims are well supported by nutritional research.

Lecithin should more properly be spoken of in the plural, for they are a group of compounds found in all fats, slightly different in each source. Soy lecithin is now the only commercial form.

Its dipolar structure makes lecithin a terrific emulsifier; one side of the molecule attracts water, the other attracts fats—very much like soap. Every cell of the body needs small amounts of lecithin as part of its membrane to control the water- and oil-soluble nutrients and wastes that go out and come in. More especially, in nerve cells, lecithin makes up much of the myelin sheath, the fatty protective sleeve around each nerve fiber. In nerve membranes, lecithin regulates the action of the "sodium pump," a sort of seesaw of charged sodium and potassium ions that carries the nerve's electrical impulses. Lecithin can function as a gentle calmative to persons deficient in it, and it has been used with some success in multiple sclerosis, in which the lecithin content of brain and nerves is drastically diminished.

Lecithin's emulsifying ability is essential for the body's adsorption of lipids (fats and oils) and the vitamins dissolved in them (A, D, E, and K). Research going back to 1943 has indicated that lecithin enables the body to use cholesterol, another essential component of the nervous and hormonal systems. Arteriosclerosis—unhealthfully high blood-cholesterol levels and deposits on the artery walls—is so complex that physicians recognize four types. Lecithin, while not useful in some cases, has dramatically lowered serum cholesterol and apparently dissolved arterial plaque in others.

Lecithin even contains two of the fatty acids it helps metabolize. In the case of soy lecithin, these are two of the essentials: linoleic and linolenic acids. Lipids cannot be digested without lecithins, but our bodies can usually synthesize enough to get by during a dietary shortage—unless the needed component parts are also missing from the table. The irony is that most natural sources of lecithin are removed from processed foods. Lecithin, comprising 1.5–3.0 percent of raw soy oil, is one of the impurities removed in the refining process; and today one cannot buy unrefined oils in most markets. Instead, the lecithin is used for candy, fire foam, Pam (a non-stick coating sprayed on frying pans for cooking), and a "food supplement" that is really a dietary restitution. Unrefined grains supply it, but the only source that remains a staple in American cuisine is the noble egg yolk.

Besides being a crucial component of semen, lecithin is essential to our sex lives in the formation and use of cholesterol; the latter is raw material for all the steroids and sterones, including the male hormones testosterone and aldosterone, the female's progesterone, and the adrenal steroids that keep us healthy and free of arthritis. Lecithin performs this function by virtue of its component, choline, an essential B vitamin. This fraction is also a precursor of acetylcholine and cholinesterase. The former is the main neurotransmitter of the brain, spinal cord, and parasympathetic nervous system; the latter is the hormone that quickly clears the synapse of acetylcholine after each nerve impulse to ready it for the next one.

Lecithin's importance to the entire nervous system may give it possibilities scarcely yet dreamed of. Doctors at the National

Institute of Mental Health clinical center in Bethesda, Maryland, recently reported that 10 grams of choline—ten times the average daily intake—produced a 17–25 percent improvement in test subjects' short-term memory of word lists. If this improvement also applies to grocery lists, thermodynamics, and umbrellas, there may soon be millions of people with a five-dollar-a-week lecithin habit. It must be stressed that the complex workings of memory are still poorly understood, and these tentative findings in no way constitute proof that lecithin has the slightest effect on real-life learning ability or retention. Still, no toxicity has ever been noted from the substance (though it is full of calories), so even the one-quarter to one-half cup daily that this 10-gram choline intake represents should cause no problems.

Lecithin is also a rich source of phosphorus, whose sex-hormone-stimulating effects are discussed on page 95.

But does it *work?* There's every reason to believe it's a temporary "aphrodisiac" for people whose tissues are deficient in it, but there's no consensus as to whether its work ends at returning a person to normal, or whether supernormal amounts may have further libido-raising effects. It certainly seemed to make me feel better, in bed and out, when I started taking a few spoons every day.

Anyone who wishes to try it must decide between the liquid and granulated forms. The liquid is more concentrated per tablespoon, but contains a fair amount of excess oil and is harder to mix. Most people find its taste and texture unbearable unless thoroughly disguised in bread or milk shakes. The granular type can be more palatably mixed with yogurt or soups, and the emulsifying properties of either can be used in salad dressings, sauces, or gravies. A few weirdos even favor its bland waxy taste straight from the bottle or mixed with a little bee pollen. Health-food booklets always suggest sprinkling it over ice cream, but I can't see many people going out of their way to mutilate thus a dish of Häagen-Dazs.

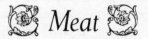# Meat

THE large per capita consumption of meat in the United States is evidence against Havelock Ellis's statement that a beefsteak is "probably as powerful a sexual stimulant as any food." Even during the centuries when upper-class English cuisine was little more than a surfeit of meats followed by assorted heavy cheeses, creams, and sweets, there is no evidence that coitus was unusually popular (although gout certainly was).

Compared with fish, all types of meat generally have less water but a great deal more fat. This gives meat a higher "satiety value," but also means it is harder to digest. If meat is to be included in a preamatory meal, care must be taken to avoid tough, juiceless cuts, thick roasts and such, for, as Norman Douglas observed in *Paneros*, "Indigestion and love will not be yoked together; they mope, each in his corner, praying for fair weather."

As a source of the phosphorus, zinc, and other minerals important to sexual health, sea flesh is a much better source than meats. But there is one substance meat supplies that fish does not: osmazome. This is usually defined as the flavorful part of meat juices, the part which is soluble in cold as well as boiling water. It is what flavors soups and sauces, forms the brown crust on roast meat, and contains the lion's share of meat's nutritional forte— free amino acids and B vitamins, especially niacin.

Osmazome was an important gustatory concept in the nineteenth century, soon after its discovery. It was considered to be the primary nutriment necessary for the French concept of health, *embonpoint* (literally, "in good shape"), a state wherein the body is filled out to its natural contours, the muscles are well defined and toned, and the skin glows with a robust color. While the nations of Western Europe were busy enslaving or exterminating the natives of Asia, Africa, and the Americas, osmazome was credited with blowing millions of puny vegetarians and fish eaters before them like chaff before the wind. Since then this theory has been questioned by considering the meat-rich diets of many obliterated hunting peoples, along with the superior weaponry and sheer blood-lust of the conquerors. The meat-equals-victory concept was given a final blow in the Vietnam War. Now many vegetarians have taken the opposite tack, asserting that a meat diet *makes* people cruel and rapacious—though the many peaceful carnivores I know make me unwilling to carry nutritional determinism that far.

Although the power of osmazome is a forgotten concept today, the substance is as prevalent as ever. It is found most abundantly in older animals (mutton and beef rather than lamb and veal) and in dark, strong-flavored meats rather than light, bland ones (goat, guinea fowl, and game rather than chicken or pork). It is the distribution of osmazome and the concentration of nutrients in certain organ meats that explain the aphrodisiac repute of the collected viands that follow.

We may as well begin with an exception to the above rule, for one of the most often served love meats in neither an organ in the usual sense nor rich in osmazome.

*Frogs' legs* taste much like chicken breasts and probably owe their place on love's table to the supposition that they would make diners more willing to spring. Whether they work or not, this recipe is a dandy:

> Toss 3 dozen frogs' legs for 5 minutes in a saucepan with 12 chopped mushrooms, 4 shallots, and 2 ounces butter. Add 1 tablespoon flour, some salt, pepper, and nutmeg, a glass of white wine, and a cup of consommé. Simmer for 10 minutes or until done. Remove the legs, thicken the sauce with 4 egg yolks mixed with 2 tablespoons heavy cream. Serve hot. For 4–6.

}}— *Game birds,* such as guinea fowl, quail, and pheasant, have been high on Cupid's list. Pigeons, partridge, turtledoves, and sparrows are included because they are said to spend more time feathering their nests than most birds. Perhaps the most famous way to give wings to love is to serve Quails Lucullus, stuffed with minced ham, shallots, goose liver, peppercorns, mixed herbs, and truffles. But the most elaborate is the *rôti sans pareil* described in A. T. Raimbault's 1814 *Le Parfait Cuisinier.* This requires an aviary of game and the dexterity of a maker of Chinese boxes. All the birds are to be boned and stuffed inside each other in the following order: anchovy paste and capers inside an olive, inside a figpecker (garden warbler), inside an ortolan, inside a lark, inside a thrush, inside a quail (wrapped in grape leaves), inside a lapwing, inside a plover, inside a partridge, inside a woodcock (rolled in bread crumbs), inside a teal, inside a guinea, inside a duck, inside a fat fowl, inside a well-hung pheasant, inside a wild goose, inside a turkey, inside a bustard. There are logistical problems in getting a lapwing inside the smaller plover, not to mention the difficulty of finding many of these birds, now driven to near extinction by recipes like this. Once these inconveniences are overcome, the whole is to be surrounded by clove-dotted onions, ham, carrots, celery, mignonette (*Reseda odorata,* gathered for its fragrant green flowers), bacon, salt and pepper, coriander seeds, garlic, and any other spices the chef fancies. It is then roasted for ten hours over a slow fire in a pan sealed with pastry.

}}— *Organ meats* have generally been more highly praised than muscle as stimulating foods. Most commonly used have been liver and kidney. These organs have approximately the same food value no matter what animal first owned them, but those from exotic game have often been supposed to give the lover a psychological advantage. Liver is even higher in phosphorus than fish and is an incredibly rich source of B vitamins and vitamin A (sometimes reaching 100,000 units per 3.5 ounces). It provides far more riboflavin and niacin per weight than any other food except bee pollen. Kidney is not so abundant as liver in any of these elements, but is still a rich and economical dish. The use of dried liver as a high-potency food was mentioned by Horace two millennia before its status as a health-food staple in America. Concentrated it is, but something happens in desiccation to make this one of the worst-tasting products ever devised. In fact, the reason many people don't like real liver is that it's too often cooked to the consistency of Frye boots.

❧— *Brains and sweetbreads* (thymus) have also been highly praised. They have less protein, vitamins, and minerals than liver, stand midway between the latter and beefsteak in fat content, and are extremely rich in  lecithin. The law of magic decrees that the best heads to put together for the sake of love are those of sparrows, since these birds were the ones harnessed to pull Aphrodite's chariot through thousands of years of myth. To test this for yourself:

> *Boil a turnip and a carrot in chick-pea broth, then slice them thinly. Boil them in half a glass of goat's milk until the liquid is nearly absorbed. Then add the brains of several male sparrows (might as well eat their mates, too, so they don't pine away with grief; sparrows mate for life) and half the amount of the gray matter of un-fledged pigeons. Sprinkle with powdered clover seeds, boil very briefly, and serve hot.*

The Romans extolled marrow as love food, perhaps because it is found in a bone. As a remedy for timidity, some Latin wit proposed leopard marrow cooked in goat's milk with lots of white pepper. Unless one could order a servant to spear the leopard, this, in an age before safari rifles, would have been the perfect kill or cure for shyness—at least with leopards.

🙢 *Snails* were Petronius's mainstay when the *Satyricon's* hero needed a restorative, and are one old-time favorite whose reputation remains in force today. They resemble fish in their digestibility and their low-fat and high-water content, but are not so rich in phosphorus and, of course, lack most of the sea minerals. Still, there are few meals that say I love you as eloquently as the milk-fed gastropods of this recipe, refined by Douglas's friend "CCC" in *Venus in the Kitchen:*

> *Feed 2–3 dozen snails on milk for 2 weeks by placing them in a covered crock and pouring a glass of milk over them each morning. When you are ready for them, soak them overnight in water with a little vinegar and salt added. Wash them, then boil for 20 minutes and remove them from their shells. Sauté with onion, garlic, rosemary, parsley, salt, and pepper. Add chopped mushrooms, ½ cup broth, a little tomato sauce, and ½ cup red wine. Finish by simmering for 15 minutes or until tender. Serves 2.*

🙢 *Genitals* of many animals have augmented the potency of men throughout the world and have even been used to give women a boost on occasion. This should come as no surprise to anyone familiar with the Doctrine of Signatures. And there is no reason to believe genital eating is not helpful. I have had several sweet "desserts" in bed after such a meal, and while I have no proof that the entrée was responsible, I did feel an uncommon urgency.

In this case common sense and experience are confirmed by the successful use of gonadotropic concentrates to elevate a diminished libido. The best of these products, like the ones distributed by the Nutri-Dyn Products Corporation (for information: 5705 Howard St., Niles, Ill. 60648), are processed at 98.6° F. to obtain the same effects as eating the glandular meat raw.

For women these preparations are made from ovarian tissue, a practice which has no historical counterpart. When Madame de Pompadour needed help to maintain her torrid love life with Louis XV, she ate, among other things, animal testicles, not ovaries. It seems there may be something to this sexual crossover, though. While ovarian hormones might make a woman more *receptive*, testosterone and related "male" hormones like aldosterone are the main mediators of sexual desire in *both* men and women. The use of testosterone-related anabolic steroids to increase muscular development among athletes has also increased desire in both sexes.

Note that there is a difference between extracted hormones and concentrates of the whole gland. Straight hormones are intended to support poorly functioning endocrines. If these organs are healthy, steady use of extracts for an added boost may disrupt the activity of the pituitary, thyroid, adrenals, or gonads, since all these glands work interdependently in a mutual feedback relationship. If your glands are healthy, there won't be much of a boost anyway, since excess testosterone is drained off in the urine and large amounts do not raise libido above a certain individual level. This hazard is probably not so great in eating animal organs, as they are less concentrated and few people cook them every day. Besides, clinical use of raw gland concentrates, which include the nucleoprotein and all other cell factors, indicates that they are absorbed by the patient's gonads, whose capacities are thereby permanently increased. How far this improvement may proceed in healthy tissue is not known.

Most often eaten have been the testicles of bulls, rams, or goats. They were highly recommended by Alexandre Dumas (*père*) in *Le grand Dictionnaire de cuisine* and are still popular in Spain, Provence, and Tuscany. They were standard fare in the private dining rooms of Gay Nineties San Francisco inns like the Poodle Dog and Maison Dorée. Calves' testicles were given a prominent place in Omero Rompini's *La Cucina dell'Amore*, while those of tigers were especially favored in the Far East when that animal was less rare than today.

The simplest and commonest method of cooking them is to remove the outer membrane and sauté them slowly on all sides in butter or oil. Sometimes a little cinnamon, clove, saffron, and lemon juice is recommended, sometimes vinegar and oil, garlic and salt. One of the fanciest surviving recipes is this bulls' balls pie of Cartolomeo Scappi, private chef to Pope Pius V:

> Boil 4 bulls' testicles in 2 cups water or chicken broth with a little salt; when tender, remove the outer membranes. Slice them, sprinkle them with white pepper, salt, cinnamon, and nutmeg. Cook a mincemeat of 1 pound lambs' kidneys, ¼–½ pound lean ham, gravy, 4 cloves garlic, and ½ teaspoon each marjoram and thyme. Line a pie dish with pastry, then cover the bottom with a slice of ham. Add a layer of the sliced testicles, then one of mincemeat, and continue in this manner until the pie is filled. Add a glass of wine before closing with the top crust. Bake in a preheated 400° F. oven about 15 minutes or until the crust is done and the filling cooked through.

Another long-standing practice, that of eating the penises of various animals, is harder to justify nutritionally, let alone ethically. It seems that little would be ingested but blood and some rather ordinary skin and vascular tissue, along with cartilage or bone in many cases. Nevertheless, scores of thousands of members have been enlisted in man's quest for potency from many (often live) animals, including whales, wolves, foxes, stags, swans, asses, bulls, and horses. The French writer Foucher d'Obsonville describes one method of preparing this vivisectionist's delight:

> The grooms lead in a stallion seven or eight years old but virile, well fed, and in good condition. They present him with a mare as though for mounting, but meanwhile restrain him so as to tease him well. Finally, at the moment when it seems to him he will be free to spring,

they adroitly pass his verge through a cord loop with a slipknot close by the belly; then, seizing the moment when the animal has its fullest erection, two men who hold the ends of the cord pull it forcefully, keeping it off the ground, and the member is torn from the body above the slipknot. By this means the fluids are retained and held in this part, which remains engorged; immediately it is washed and cooked with various aphrodisiac aromatics and spices.

A dish of sow's vulva, mercifully taken after the animal is slaughtered, was probably the food stimulant in which the Romans had most confidence. Apicius, editor of the only surviving Roman cookbook, gives half a dozen recipes for this transsexual aphrodisiac, and Horace, Pliny, and Martial all accord it the greatest honor. The following recipe is close to the way the Greeks cooked it and allegedly helped keep health-food pioneer Bernarr MacFadden potent well into his eighties:

> Marinate one cleaned sow's vulva in ½–¾ cup white wine in which a chopped onion, a chopped celery stalk, and ½ teaspoon each fennel seeds, peppercorns, ginger, saffron, and salt have been cooked. After a few hours, dredge the vulva [try not to wince] in flour and brown it in a skillet with a little olive oil. Strain the marinade and add it gradually to the pan to keep the meat from scorching. Add lemon or orange juice to taste just before serving.

⫸ *Other meats* allegedly aphrodisiac are the horny goat, emblem of Pan and the Satyrs; wild ass; steak tartare, to retain the vitamin E lost in cooking; goose or goose tongues; saddle of wild boar (roasted three hours in a pastry-covered dish with cinnamon, cloves, coriander and fennel seeds, ginger, nutmeg, pepper, ham, white wine, and juniper berries); and the tail of young crocodile.

In China the meat of the *black chow,* a stocky breed of dog, still enjoys a certain acclaim, although its most famous proponent is now dead. From about 1900 to his death in about 1935, "the general with the three long legs," Chang Chung-ch'ang, ate chow every day. To this dish he credited the size and hardness that led to his best-known nickname, 72-cannon Chang, derived from his penile dimensions—the equivalent of a stack of 72 silver dollars.

}◆⸺ *Skink* and *hippomanes*—the final two morsels in our amatory abattoir—belong to the same class of presumably hormone-rich tissues as testicles and ovaries, but they are more difficult to obtain. The skink is a small lizard (*Lacerta scincus* or *Scincus officinalis*). We first know of its use from the writings of the Greeks and Romans, but it must have been known as a sexual food far earlier in its native East Africa and Arabia. Large quantities of its dried flesh were exported from Cairo to Venice and Marseilles; it was a fairly common delicacy among many Arab tribes as late as the 1930s, but I am not sure how well it is surviving today. One variety is reportedly eaten in the Antilles under the name of *mabouiha* or *brochet terrestre.* The entire animal is considered inflammatory, and the most often recorded recipe calls for filleting the flesh along the backbone, dipping it in beaten egg seasoned with herbs, and frying it in olive oil. But the most powerful part of the lizard's body is apparently the genital tissue. According to Dr. Nicolas Venette's *Tableau de l'amour conjugal,* it "works wonders in inciting a man to love" when it is dried, powdered, and drunk in sweet wine.

There is some confusion concerning the identity of hippomanes (from the Greek, literally, "horse madness"), because Vergil describes it as a "clammy poison" that flows from the vaginas of mares during the spring rutting season. Most other classical references, including a different one by Vergil, refer to the fleshy caul or excrescence, about the size of a fig, which is found on the head of a newborn colt and which the mother eats before giving suck to her foal. To be used by humans it must be snatched from the animal almost at the very moment of birth.

Hippomanes seems to have the same effect on stallions that it is claimed to have on human studs. Pausanias records that the sculptor Phormis Menalius once made a horse of brass into which he had mixed hippomanes while the metal was still molten. Though the replica was a poor one and had no tail, every spring stallions had to be discouraged by the whip from their frenzied attempts to copulate with it. Would-be experimenters are on their own here, however, for use of hippomanes seems to have died out with the fall of Rome, and no detailed recipes have survived.

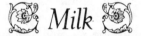

## Milk

MILK was often mentioned in pastoral poetry as the food of pretty shepherdesses, but among us it is seldom mentioned in the same breath with sex, being more associated with kiddies, old maids, and milquetoast. This state of affairs is puzzling, since milk should be a part of everyone's first sexual or quasi-sexual experience. Maybe our milk aversion can be traced to the decline in breast feeding in recent generations and the substitution of sterile formula and a neoprene teat for a real nipple with genetically matched elixir of mother.

Many people in later life find the liquid indigestible and question whether we were meant to drink the milk of other species long after our own weaning. Lactose intolerance, an inability to digest milk sugar, is the problem most often cited. Judging by its high rate among adult blacks and Ashkenazi Jews, lack of the proper intestinal enzymes may be genetically determined, and some people may indeed not be meant to drink milk.

On the other hand, some nutrition-oriented doctors have found that if milk drinking is continued from childhood, the body's ability to produce the digestive enzymes remains into adulthood. In a lifetime of successful practice based on Hippocrates' approach of healing with food before resorting to drugs, the late Dr. Harry Bieler found that raw milk (certified from healthy, inspected cows) was easily digested by most people who could not stomach the pasteurized variety. He concluded that heat processing so changes this most delicate food as to make it detrimental to many people, but argued that raw cow's or goat's milk—drunk slowly and between, not with, meals—is generally the most easily digested food of all.

Whether or not his conclusions gain wide acceptance, milk is the best natural source of calcium and riboflavin (vitamin $B_2$), and its quota of usable protein is matched only by that of eggs. Even more relevant to our study is milk's zinc content. Newborn animals require large amounts of zinc, and colostrum (first milk secretion) has been found to be phenomenally high in this mineral, up to 900 milligrams per 100 grams in nursing mothers. Zinc levels in milk at all stages of secretion vary with the amounts in the mother's diet. Human diets today are often so deficient that some babies are better off—from the zinc standpoint—with milk from a cow than from their own mother. Cow's milk, even from animals grazing on grass from zinc-deficient soils, is the best source, except for seafood.

It is time for a reevaluation of milk's potential as a sexually fortifying food. A few nutritionists, like Dr. Bieler and Paavo Airola, have already called for a reconsideration, but at the moment the only ones to agree are such farsighted ancients as Shaykh Nefzawi, who loved camel's milk with honey, and Avicenna, who claimed chameleon's milk to be a potent love drink.

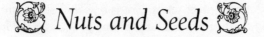
SEEDS are little legacies—everything young embryos need to set up in business for themselves. They contain respectable amounts of all vital nutrients: proteins, vitamins, minerals, carbohydrates, and oils. They also contain enzymes and growth hormones which, while not usually the same as those in human bodies, can be easily rearranged to suit our needs. German nutrition researcher Dr. Bela Pater has written that the plant hormones in pumpkin seeds, for example, seem to support human hormone production and that the incidence of prostate trouble is near zero in areas where pumpkin seeds are regularly included in the diet.

Half the weight of most nuts and seeds is oil, and most varieties are rich in polyunsaturated fatty acids. They are good sources of lecithin, vitamin E, and the B vitamins essential to cell respiration—the body's fuel-burning process. They are exceptionally rich in minerals, including magnesium, potassium, phosphorus, zinc, and many trace elements—such as manganese, molybdenum, and vanadium—needed for various catalyzing enzymes in all cells. Zinc is a crucial ingredient of several of the secretions that form semen, and most nuts are good sources of it, although lower than milk, seafood, liver, and whole wheat.

Most nuts are also rich in protein, but since they are all deficient in at least one of the amino acids essential to humans, they need to be combined with each other or with other sources before their protein can be well utilized. All except the starchy types, like chestnuts, are best eaten raw; roasting lowers the digestibility of their protein, accelerates the rancidification of their oils, and destroys their enzymes. Besides, the oil and salt usually added are nutritional extras we are better off without.

Seeds and nuts are an integral part of any balanced diet, but there is no sexual advantage to be gained from emphasizing them at the expense of other foods. Nor is one kind significantly better than another. Butternuts, peanuts, pine nuts, and sunflower seeds are highest in protein. Unshelled sesame seeds have five times as much calcium as any other seed or nut. Brazil nuts and pumpkin and sunflower seeds lead in phosphorus; pumpkin, sesame, and pistachio have the most iron; pine and sunflower are tops in thiamine content; almonds are best for riboflavin; sunflower seeds for magnesium; and peanuts have far more niacin than any other nut. All in all, mixed nuts are best. Old bedtime nut recipes generally take account of this fact. The Arabs and Indians usually mingled their pine nuts, pistachios, and almonds. An old English favorite called for chestnuts soaked in muscatel, then boiled with pistachios and pignolias (pine nuts), but this one probably owed more to the other ingredients: cubeb peppers, rocket seed, cinnamon, and satyrion.

Only one nut has achieved individual fame as an aphrodisiac. This is the huge seed of the sea coconut (*Lodoicea seychellarum*). Over a foot in diameter and weighing up to fifty pounds, this nut at one end bears a striking resemblance to a woman's hips and crotch; that is why the seed's genus name was taken from the loveliest of the daughters of King Priam of Troy—Laodice.

Before the age of exploration *coco de mer* was known to Europeans and most Asians only by the empty husks of germinated nuts found floating in the sea. These shells became famed not only as an aphrodisiac, but as a universal antidote. Since it was thought they could neutralize any poison, cups made from the shell were in great demand among kings. In many monarchies, a common citizen found in possession of a *coco de mer* shell had his hands cut off. The ivorylike interior layer was considered the best part to use for a love potion, especially mixed with coral, ebony, or stag's horn.

In 1640 John Parkinson's *Theatrum Botanicum* became the

first Western source to debunk the belief that these trees, never yet seen by white men, grew underwater, the protruding tops guarded by ravenous griffins that ate approaching ships. It was 1768 before exploration of the Seychelles in the Indian Ocean disclosed the world's only sea coconut forests, where these majestic palms send their rigid trunks one hundred feet into the air and live for eight hundred years. Today their much reduced population remains only on the Seychelle Islands of Praslin and Curieuse under government protection, bearing eloquent testimony to the psychological power of rarity.

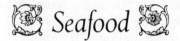

# Seafood

*Serve me my favorite dish—Fish.*
—THOMAS "FATS" WALLER

ONE of the most prevalent Greek myths has it that Aphrodite was born from the foam that gathered around the genitals of the sky god Uranus when his son Cronus cut them off and threw them into the salt sea. On her mother's side she was descended from Thetis, creator of the universe and mother of all life as ruler of the sea.

Like the fatal mermaid she later became, Aphrodite beckons us down through the foam to the origin of desire, into the young sea of the Cambrian period, when the first testicular sac—a sort of pocket-husband like Uranus's disembodied genitals—developed on the side of an organism akin to the modern *Cirripedia* (barnacles) and the first division into sexes occurred among multicellular animals.

The similarity of blood to seawater is one of the commonplaces of our own scientific mythology. Sodium and chloride ions are the sea's main inorganic components, with traces of magnesium, potassium, calcium, and sulfates. Of course the blood must carry myriad hormones and nutrients in the business of living, but it still reflects a heroic attempt by the body to give every cell an interior ocean like the one it came from. The main elements present in blood that are not found in such high concentrations in seawater are phosphorus and zinc. Luckily for us, most sea creatures and some land plants concentrate these atoms in their tissues.

Aphrodite's meats are richer in phosphorus, potassium, and zinc than land meats and most other foods. For example, 100 grams (about 3.5 ounces) of cooked eggs supply roughly 200 milligrams of phosphorus. The same amount of the best sirloin yields 250; chicken a little less. Most seafoods have at least this much. Bluefish and shad hover around the 300 mark, while salmon and some kinds of fish roe top 400 milligrams per 100 grams. Levels of most amino acids and other minerals are about the same in sea protein as in land sources, but even the fattyest fish have less fat than lean meat, and although fish oils are harder to digest, they provide much more vitamin A. Seafood is a much better source of zinc for semen and the iodine needed for thyroid hormones to regulate energy levels. Oysters, it turns out, are a uniquely potent source of zinc, providing about ten times more per weight than any other food.*

As far as I know there have been no chemical analyses of sea foam, but at least we can better appreciate why the ocean's progeny have been sacred to the queen of love in all ages. The following survey is by no means the complete fish story; if you get lost, remember the password: swordfish.

## ---⊰{ CAVIAR }⊱---

Right at the womb of the matter is caviar, the pearl of the kitchen, essence of fish, with the power to send its devotees at one gulp back to the happy spawning ground of evolutionary regression.

Roe is fine from any fish, but when we speak of caviar we

---

*From exceptionally well-fed cows, the zinc level of milk may reach one-third that of oysters (see Milk, page 55).

usually mean the roe of the virgin sturgeon, the "very fine fish"
that inspired an unknown rhymer to tell how

*I gave caviar to my girl friend,*
*She was a virgin tried and true;*
*Ever since she had the caviar,*
*There ain't nothing she won't do!*

He probably spent a week's salary on his date that night, and
maybe she originated the gallant lady's rejoinder for such occasions: "You pay for the caviar and the rest of the evening is on
me." Caviar is worth it—that's the consensus of the monied few
who blew a $10-million wad on the world's 300,000 pounds of
available caviar in 1978. Few foods have the language of wealth
arguing its merits so persuasively. Prices and supplies fluctuate
with rumors of sturgeon extinction, just like oil (industrial pollution and gradual evaporation of its sea now threaten the most valued variety in its native Caspian). But those who can afford the
current $250 a pound for the best malosol ("little salt") beluga
have always shown they would buy ten times the available stock.
Bidding for the supply is so keen that for the past several years
Russia, unable to meet its own demand, has leaked a rumor that
the Soviet Union Laboratory of Physics has devised a palatable
formula for imitation caviar, apparently in an attempt to drive the
price down. So far no one has shown much interest, and the ersatz
has not materialized. But Iranian exports have fallen off drastically
since the Islamic revolution, so perhaps a substitute will be marketed after all.

Alexander the Great got a taste for sturgeon roe from Darius
and passed it by way of the Ptolemys to a long line of Roman emperors, who often had the live fish relayed in huge tubs by teams
of runners from the Caspian to the Capital. Caviar will remain
primarily a king's appetizer, but many delicatessens, epitomized
by New York's Caviarteria, now cater to a market of occasional
splurgers.

One hundred grams of granular caviar contains 355 milligrams of phosphorus, 276 of calcium, smatterings of most known vitamins, and 27 grams of protein. (Pressed caviar is slightly more concentrated, but also saltier and less esteemed by gourmets.) It is these ingredients that make it a bona fide sexual food, which sexologist Dr. William J. Robinson recommended in cases of nutritionally reversible impotence. Its extremely high sodium content, however, makes it a poor choice for heart patients. Robinson's advice would have been easy to follow less than a century ago, when sturgeon were so plentiful in North America that free caviar on bread was complimentary with a glass of nickel beer in many saloons.

Whatever your means, there is no approved method of eating the eggs you have scored, except that they should not touch metal and thus absorb its taste. Bygone Casanovas and Pompadours loved such recipes as Harlots' Eggs (one tablespoon each of anchovy paste, chives, and pimiento, and a squeeze of lemon juice mixed with one-half cup caviar), but those who can afford an addiction usually prefer it straight on thin toast, barely highlighted by lemon or pepper, with champagne or vodka on the side.

## --⊷{ FISH }⊷--

Among the Greeks, Asclepiades advised· "For a meal with a courtesan, a purchase is to be made of three large and ten small fish and twenty-four prawns." The Roman bucolic poet Ausonius devoted 150 lines to the exciting fish of the Moselle in his charming pastoral poem of the same name. English balladeer Thomas Jordan advised that "fish dinners will make a lass spring like a flea."

When Catherine the Great desperately needed to marshal support by producing an heir to her crown, which she had failed to do by her husband, she called on a guard and a fish. She ordered some caviar, a huge sturgeon, and a fine officer named Saltikoff and soon had a prospect for her legacy.

This wide cross-cultural agreement has led many observers to wonder why the Church perversely made fish the primary food of its monks and fast days (to make chastity as much a test of will as possible?). The ancient Egyptians more sensibly *forbade* seafood to their celibate priests. Perhaps this deliberate folly originated in the period when the Christian fathers enhanced their faith's popularity by incorporating many of the outward trappings of pagan ritual into their own. Easter is generally held to have descended from universally practiced fertility rites of spring, presided over by the goddess of dawn and the sea—the Germanic Eastre, equivalent of the Phoenician Astarte and Babylonian Ishtar. The symbolic fecundation of the earth was usually renewed every Friday (the day of Freya, the German Aphrodite), after a meal of sacred fish.

Nicolas Venette, oddly enough, ascribes the power of fish to their high water content, possibly an oblique reference to their easy digestibility or to the seawater-blood-semen connection. Whether we believe in water or phosphorus or zinc, there has been no lack of popular experimentation to prove the point.

## --◄ EELS ►--

Eels are valued above scaly fish in some cultures, as in classical Greece, where Aristophanes built one of his antiwar comedies, *The Acharnians,* around a love for the elvers of Lake Copais so strong that citizens abandoned their own government to sue for a separate peace with Boeotia.

The eel has been the phallic stand-in for the snake in some Pacific areas where snakes are rare, and they have been given feminine meaning in expressions like "She's the eel's hips," from our Roaring Twenties. In most areas where they are valued as food, they are thought to have an exceptionally enlivening effect on sexual mores. For American, European, and Mediterranean eels, perhaps this is because they journey thousands of miles to mate in the energy-charged waters of the Bermuda Triangle's Sargasso Sea. Then again, the eel's fat levels and concentrations of vitamins A and D (far higher than any other fish) may be responsible. Maybe eels' resistance to pollution (due to oxygen needs lower than other fish) simply make them livelier these days.

Whichever is the case, I find eels even more delicious than most scaly fish, more filling, and conducive to a more pronounced feeling of tightness and eagerness. And the best dish I've come across is this delicious matelote with raisins given by Raymond Sokolov in a recent issue of *Natural History* magazine (Vol. 87, no. 5, May 1978, p. 100), very much like a dish that used to amuse Aristophanes' audiences.

*Melt 3 tablespoons butter in a heavy saucepan. Add 4 white onions, 2 quartered carrots, 2 cloves garlic and ⅓ cup flour; stir over medium-low heat about 10 minutes until the vegetables are coated with golden flour. Stir in 1 cup water, 3 cups dry red wine, and 2 tablespoons cognac; add a bouquet garni (½ stalk celery, 2 sprigs fresh parsley and thyme, and a bay leaf), 1 clove, and salt and pepper. Bring to a boil, cover, and simmer for 45 minutes.*

*Melt 3 more tablespoons butter in a skillet and quickly brown 1½ to 2 pounds cleaned, skinned eels cut into 2-inch pieces. Remove eels and keep warm. Add ½ pound mushrooms, both chopped and whole, to the butter remaining in the skillet, add 2 tablespoons lemon juice, and sauté for 5 minutes.*

*Plump ½ cup golden raisins by pouring boiling water on them. Let stand for 3 minutes, then drain.*

*Strain the vegetable-herb sauce into a clean saucepan and simmer the eel pieces in it until they flake easily— 10–30 minutes.*

*Fry 6 small triangles decrusted bread in 2 tablespoons butter and drain on paper towels. Top the eels with some of the sauce (serve the rest on the side) to which*

the raisins and mushrooms have been added at the last minute. Garnish the dish with the whole mushrooms and bread. Serves 4.

## --◄ FISH SAUCE ►--

Roman cooks made frequent use of a sauce they called *liquamen* or *garum*. It was as essential to their cuisine as soy sauce is to Oriental chefs. In fact, it bore some resemblance to soy sauce, except that it was made from anchovies, mackerel, and the entrails of other fish packed in salt and allowed to decompose in the sun for a few days. Details are unclear, but it seems that liquamen was the liquid first pressed out of this mass, while garum was made from it by adding various spices. Liquamen was probably very similar to the *nuoc-mam* sauce of Southeast Asia. The supposedly lascivious nature of the Annamese (Vietnamese) was blamed by nineteenth-century Western travelers on nuoc-mam's high concentrations of sodium, phosphorus, and other fish minerals.

Many Americans got a taste of nuoc-mam during the Vietnam War, but, as one of its minor tragedies, the conflict produced a marked decline in the quality of the sauce. Today Asian neighborhood markets in the United States sometimes carry nuoc-mam from Thailand or a Filipino liquamen called *patis*. The following recipe for scallop sausages is given partly because it tastes great and partly as an example of how garum was used by the Romans. It comes from the second- or third-century cookbook attributed to the first-century gourmet Apicius.

> Mix minced scallops with some flour and beaten eggs, season well with pepper, wrap in a caul, and fry. Serve with a fish sauce made like a mayonnaise from mashed hard-boiled egg yolks, dates, honey, lovage, cumin, onion, origan [marjoram], mustard, vinegar, garum, and oil. [Worcestershire sauce mixed with anchovy paste can substitute for garum in a pinch.]

Two Chinese soups enjoy lively reputations as love stimulants. Shark's fin (*sha ch'i*) soup, considered the lesser of the two, is made not from the whole fins, but only from the yellow cartilage after the skin, bone, and meat have been removed by parboiling. In the soup, the cartilage becomes gelatinous and serves as a sponge for the flavors of other ingredients—usually chicken and/or ham, garlic, scallions, and ginger.

Bird's nest (*yen wo*) soup is a similar setting for the nests of the *Collocalia* genus of swifts that dwell along the cliffs of the China coast and several islands in the Indian Ocean. It used to be thought that the soup's aphrodisiac effect was due to quantities of phosphorus in fish spawn and iodine in seaweed used to hold the nests together. Now that it has been learned that the nests are made almost entirely of the birds' especially sticky saliva, this explanation has died. I have found no analysis of the bird spittle, but, judging from my own lack of reaction, I see no reason to believe either of these concoctions is any more stimulating than gelatin. Both are tasteless themselves, although the soup around them can be delicious. Shark's fin and bird's nest can be bought in most Chinatown markets. The best nests are a silvery white with no feathers. Beware of cheap imitations made from old nests boiled down with agar, although I'm not sure what difference the fraud would make in the result.

--◄{ *TREPANG* }►--

Another Asian favorite is the slow-moving, phallic-looking creature gathered from coral reefs and variously known as the sea cucumber, sea slug, trepang, *oh nyeow sam*, or *bêche-de-mer*. These are any of several species of *Holothuria*, a few inches to a few feet long, black, brown, green, or reddish, and smooth or covered with blunt prickles. They are found in equatorial oceans throughout the world but are usually ignored as food outside of Asia. Their signature is their amusing habit of filling themselves with water in a manner resembling an erection when they are touched.

Trepang are available throughout Asia and in some Oriental groceries in the United States. For commercial use they are usually split and eviscerated (their stomachs are filled with gritty little shells of the tiny marine life they eat), then sun-dried or smoked. One method of cooking them, popular in Korea, involves soaking them overnight, then slicing them and frying with onions, scallions, garlic, ginger, and hot green chili peppers. The dish is washed down with beer. I have to rate this one of the least effective aphrodisiacs I have ever tried, with no taste but smoke and peppers and a texture of Goodyear radials. A more palatable recipe calls for boiling them for several hours until they become gelatinous, then grinding them and adding to soups.

---˦ *FUGU* ˦---

One of the world's most reliably potent aphrodisiacs enjoys a certain vogue in Japan, but I have no intention of including it in my research until I am a good deal more desperate than now, perhaps suffering from a terminal illness. I am speaking of fugu, a species of puffer fish whose flesh is eaten raw as sashimi and whose testicular fluid is mixed with a cup of hot sake and drunk.

The problem with fugu is that its ovaries, liver, and certain other organs contain a deadly nerve poison called tetradoxin. By Japanese law it can only be prepared by licensed fugu chefs, and the surgical skill required is such that only about 30 percent of all candidates get their certificate. At unknown number of Japanese and Western visitors take their chances each year. If the cook has made a mistake, it becomes evident within minutes as the diner drops his glass, collapses, stops breathing, and soon dies. There is no known antidote, and an average of three hundred people get the last thrill of their lives from fugu every year. It is not yet known whether the neurotoxin and the aphrodisiac component are different compounds or the same one in different concentrations; to my knowledge no attempts have been made to separate the two.

Octopus, shrimp, trepang, fugu, terrapin, crab, crayfish, cod—all have their advocates, from the Romans who called starfish and remora the most aphrodisiac of all to Henry Fielding and his cunning digression on lobsters in *Tom Jones*. But the most popular and effective seafood of all are hard-shelled shellfish—oysters, clams, mussels, etc. The anonymous author of the ballad "Grand Affair of Eating" sums it up in this couplet:

> *Eat Beef or Pye-crust if you'd serious be;*
> *Your Shell-fish raises* Venus *from the Sea.*

Huge refuse heaps of shells at prehistoric sites around the world testify that the preferred type was usually oysters. This choice may represent an intuitive "knowledge" of their richness in zinc as well as their legendary digestibility. Casanova as a rule breakfasted on fifty on the half shell every day and was fond of playing his "oyster game" in seduction maneuvers. This consisted of jestingly talking his target into eating oysters from his own lips, allowing himself to drop some of the juice on her "alabaster spheres," and feeling obliged to lick them clean, all to the accompaniment of background music, amorous verse, and tales of his prowess.

Oysters are mostly protein, minerals, and water, and they are so easily digested that experienced eaters sometimes down a gross or more as an appetizer without diminishing their zest for the meal ahead. Long aware of this fact, Brillat-Savarin once tested its limits while he was director of the commissary of the revolutionary directorate. He invited a certain Laperte to dine with him, a man who often complained that he could never get his fill of oysters. The gourmet professor kept pace with him through the third dozen, but then sat in ever more impatient dismay as Laperte began to hit his stride at the *thirty-second* dozen, looking as though he wished the maid could open the shells faster. The host finally halted the experiment to get to the second course, which his guest attacked "with the vigor and polish of a man finishing a long fast."

But the best oyster story I have ever heard concerns the young bride whose tale was first printed in Paul Haines' "A Critique of Pure Bawdry." Having some fears about her fiancé's shyness, she sought help from her friend the oysterman. He told her to have the wedding supper at his place and leave the rest to him. He served them each a dozen of his plumpest specimens. Seeing her the next day and asking how it had gone, he received her profuse thanks but was told, "Alas, six of them didn't work."

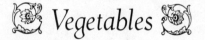 *Vegetables*

THERE was a reason why, as kids, we never finished the spinach and slipped the broccoli in our pockets to avoid eating it. No matter how essential they are to our health, vegetables are watery, seldom sweet, and, at least the way they're cooked for babies, pastelike. They have never been banned for leading to sin. Except for the legumes, most have too much water and too little protein to qualify. But several exceptions lustily prove the rule. And, especially as salads, with each plant reinforcing the other's vitamin and mineral contributions, vegetables make all the richer foods more easily absorbed and more effective.

Where this fact has not been appreciated or the climate has been too cold to grow vegetables, people have suffered greatly from gout, arthritis, and kidney ailments fostered by overreliance on meat. Elsewhere, landowners have traditionally valued their gardens immensely. Contrary to popular belief, the Greeks and Romans ate a predominantly vegetarian diet; meat was mostly for the rich. And even among the aristocracy, a finely landscaped garden of at least four or five acres was an essential possession, giving its owner a tranquil place to meditate as well as good side dishes.

In England, where vegetable cultivation first became important in Elizabethan times, the English borrowed the Continental practice of planting the garden as a sort of picture, arranging the herbs in geometric designs or in the form of a love knot. Choice of crops was often based on aphrodisiac reputation. Most gardens included the famed artichoke; the phallic asparagus, carrot, and parsnip; the flatulent bean; and various onions. Rabelais enumerated the sexy plants he liked in his salads: "rocket, tarragon, cresses, parsley, rampions [the evening primrose, *Oenothera biennis*, a former garden favorite used for its young spring leaves and radishlike root], poppy [probably for the seeds or petals of the red poppy, *Papaver rhoeas*], and celery." The American Colonists, besides finding they could grow bigger carrots than in the Old World, favored aromatic dill, chervil, and spearmint. They used nutrient-rich dandelion as a medicine for impotence and grew periwinkle for its allegedly lust-inciting leaves. Three ounces of young dandelion leaves give an incredible 12,000 units of vitamin A, more than even kale or parsley. The periwinkle potion is harder to explain, since its leaves have not been so thoroughly analyzed. Most herbals list it only as an astringent diarrhea remedy and a sedative.

Most vegetables figure in an occasional bit of love lore, some with good reason, some with none. Popeye always got Olive Oyl after downing his child-indoctrinating spinach, supposedly because of its high iron content. But spinach is no richer in iron than many other foods, and adsorption of much of its food value is blocked by the oxalic acid it contains.

Watercress and garden cress (peppergrass) have a long history in aphrodisiac folklore, probably because of their hot taste and because both are good sources of vitamin A, potassium, and calcium. Cress and nettle seed (with its burning oil) was one of the preparations most widely used among the Romans. Ovid, Martial, Columella, and Petronius testify to popular belief that cress is *impudica*, "shameless." For impotence the Roman doctor Marcellus Empiricus prescribed doses of 3 scruples (⅛ ounce or almost 4 grams) of each of the following: cress, sweet red onion, pine nuts, and Indian nard (spikenard). The cookbook author Apicius avers that boiled onions with pine nuts, cress juice, and pepper is an effective love stimulant.

The sweet potato is one of the very few vegetables that sometimes achieves a balance of enough essential amino acids to make it a worthy protein food by itself, though not all varieties do so. Thus there is some reason for its reputation among New World Indian tribes and its occasional use in American slang as a term of endearment.

A little harder to explain is the former use of lettuce as an aphrodisiac in German brothels. All types except iceberg are fairly high in potassium and vitamin A, but otherwise lettuce doesn't even have the phallic assets of Belgian endive, once used as a love charm by young fräuleins.

Another puzzler is the radish. It was one of the favorite vegetables of the ancient Egyptians. Many tons of the roots fed the pyramid work gangs. A papyrus of about 500 B.C. names the root as a sure aphrodisiac when eaten with honey, and other eras attributed the same powers to its gas-producing properties. French poet Claude Bigothier went so far as to compose a long *Raphorum Encomium* ("Eulogy of Radishes") in 1540.

In the Orient, the oversized, penis-shaped *daikon*, pickled or fresh, sometimes weighing a hundred pounds, is even more esteemed by lovers. But unless ancient ones were different from today's, or they contain some factor yet unknown, radishes are one of the least nutritious of vegetables. They provide significant amounts only of the ubiquitous potassium and are 95 percent water.

The tomato is another aphrodisiac mistake. Long cultivated throughout tropical and subtropical America, this Andean native was first brought to Europe by Cortes. For centuries thereafter it was called the love apple, probably because of a semantic mix-up. In one version the Italians called them *pomi dei Moro* ("Moor's apples"), since Spaniards were colloquially known as Moors. This was then misheard by the French as *pommes d'amour*. Another version has a similar corruption coming from the Italian *pomo d'oro* ("golden apple"), and a third tale simply says that Sir Walter Raleigh, hoping to excite Queen Elizabeth in his favor, said they were apples of love when he first showed them to her.

Perhaps the tomato's close botanical relationship to mandrake and other daturas added fuel to the imaginary fire; it certainly led to centuries of popular belief that the food was poisonous. The same thing happened to potatoes and eggplants. In any event, no matter how scarlet or succulent, vine-ripened reds (or the even sweeter golden ones) are merely the juiciest of summer refreshers. Their aphrodisiac power survives today mainly in the universal slang, "hot tomato," for a woman of warmth.

Many vegetables deserve a more prominent place on the bedside table than the preceding ones, and we will shortly take a look at the most esteemed. But first I would like to plead for the addition of an as yet unrecognized food to our aphrodisiac pantry—the red bell pepper. It has no overwhelming nutritional qualifications, although two medium pods provide a hefty 4,500 units of vitamin A and 200 milligrams of vitamin C. Its appeal lies in a sweet insouciance that only fresh-picked corn can match, a juicy red stain on the lips that invites a kiss or ten, and the form and color of the lovelorn human heart itself.

### ---◖ ARTICHOKES ◗---

"The artichoke," observed Richard Armour, "is the only vegetable of which there is more after it has been eaten," adding that a dentist would be able to identify a felon by the teeth marks on discarded leaves if artichokes had been eaten at the scene of a crime. Perhaps because it is the only common vegetable whose nourishing part is its reproductive organ, or flower, the artichoke has long been given a prominent place in love's kitchen.

The ancient Mediterranean cultures thought this edible thistle gave its eaters an extra boost for the pleasures of the bed. Roman aristocrats consumed large quantities, both of the globe artichoke and its close relative, the cardoon, whose leaf stalks are eaten instead of its buds. Pliny alone dissented, calling artichokes "monstrous productions of the earth" and noting that animals won't touch them.

Catherine de Médicis followed common knowledge by feeding them to her lovers, and their reputation was echoed by Dr. Nicolas Venette, whose seventeenth-century marriage manual attributed "much semen and vigor" to the artichoke. Of course, he may have been unduly partial to a vegetable closer to the French heart than most. The good doctor had no doubt encountered the proverb that says artichokes are good for women ("when men eat them") and often heard the classic pitch of Parisian market vendors:

> Artichokes! Artichokes!
> Heats the body and the spirit.
> Heats the genitals.

Some types grow enormous heads three or four feet in diameter, and the large, succulent ones are often eaten raw in Europe, seasoned with salt and pepper. Steamed or straight, large or small, they all have approximately the same nutritional value—a little calcium and phosphorus, more potassium, and traces of B vitamins. The caloric content can vary widely, from 8 to 44 for a 3.5 ounce globe.

As an aphrodisiac, asparagus is often dismissed today as mere symbolism, a vibrant stalk signifying much but delivering nothing serviceable to the gonads. Its symbolism gains a new level of meaning when, in the best cooking method, those trim little soldiers stand upright in one rigid phalanx, bound together, heads held high, ready for the sacrifice, about to enter the boiling caldron and become a divinity of a vegetable course. You must remember, by the way, to immerse your mercenaries only waist-deep, so as not to cook the spears too soft or the shafts too hard.

Asparagus contains several nutrients that give it some claim as an extremely healthful food, if not a true aphrodisiac. It provides more protein per calorie than most vegetables, but being 93 percent water, it has little of either. Its moderate amounts of vitamin A, potassium, and calcium help maintain the body's energy level, and its phosphorus helps make sex hormones.

Asparagus contains aspartic, the amino acid used in the process of transamination by which nitrogen from excess protein is removed from the body. The vegetable also provides the amino acid asparagine, needed by all cells for their elimination of wastes. Asparagine in the diet acts as a diuretic, and its urinary stimulation can produce a vague excitation in nearby genital organs. These two nutrients also take out ammonia circulating in the blood, which helps prevent fatigue. This may be why Culpeper's *Herbal* of 1654 prescribes asparagus for gout and strangury. Culpeper also claims that a brew of asparagus roots, boiled in wine and taken first thing in the morning several days running, "stirreth up bodily lust in man or woman, whatever some have written to the contrary."

Asparagus once had the virtue of rarity going for it, but Thomas Jefferson and other growers helped introduce it to plebeian markets by starting new beds (the crux of cultivation is readying the bed) from seed-grown greenhouse stock. A couple of generations earlier, Madame de Pompadour had devised the following aristocratic recipe for her "little suppers":

> *Cook 2–3 pounds of asparagus sticks by plunging them into boiling water. Slice them obliquely towards the tips into pieces no bigger than the little finger. Take only the choicest sections and, keeping them hot, allow them to drain while the sauce is being prepared.*
>
> *Knead together 10 grams of flour and a lump of butter, a good pinch of powdered nutmeg and the yolks of 2 eggs diluted with 4 spoonsful of water acidulated with lemon juice. After cooking this sauce, drop in the asparagus tips and serve in a covered casserole.*

It is possible that this recipe reached La Pompadour indirectly from Arab sources, for *The Perfumed Garden* contains a sketchy but similar one. Sir Richard F. Burton translates it as "boiled asparagus, fried in fat," but the end result will be more appetizing if we make it "blanched and sautéed." The dish is then topped with a sauce of egg yolk and ground spices.

What bananas were to Josephine Baker, asparagus was to the nyloned lovelies of belle époque French magazines like *La Vie Parisienne* and *Le Rire.* They continued a symbolic tradition that stems from the Phoenicians, Greeks, and Romans by way of Rabelais's "uniterminal, intercrural [between the legs] asparagus stalk."

Brillat-Savarin tells a tale of an enormous asparagus, many inches around, found growing in the garden of Monseigneur Courtois de Quincey, Bishop of Belley. The cleric had a local cutler make a special knife for the specimen, and when it looked ripe, he tried to cut it, only to find it was made of wood. At first he did not know how to take the prank, played by a subordinate priest who had carved the tip and stealthily raised it a little each night. But then the bishop joined the general mirth, forgave the devout asparaginist, and exhibited his handiwork in the drawing room. But even such art has not bested nature in the matter of asparagus size, for the Roman emperors sometimes dined on stalks twelve feet tall brought by their legionnaires from North Africa's Getulian plains.

## ⸺⋇ CELERY ⋇⸺

Like asparagus, celery owes its meager aphrodisiac reputation to a confusion of the kidneys with the gonads. Celery's sweeter cousin, Florence fennel (*finocchio*), is made into an esteemed love soup in parts of Italy, and like fennel, celery juice is such a strong diuretic that it is often forbidden to persons with acute urinary problems. Both have a fine balance of sodium and potassium ions for our nerves, and their effects are greater when left untrimmed, with the full bush of celery's pungent leaves and Florence's feathery tendrils intact.

John Lust's *Herb Book* lists the yellow oil distilled from celeriac (knob celery) as a remedy to restore potency after illness, but only a few sexologists have termed the stalk a stimulant. Its heyday in boudoir kitchenettes was eighteenth-century France. As an upper-class luxury, celery became haute cuisine when rumor had it that Madame de Pompadour relied on the following famous soup to enflame her aging king. Nevertheless, her recipe probably owes more to the garnish than to the main ingredient:

> *Chop, scald, and drain 1 stalk celery. Heat it in a saucepan with 1 tablespoon butter, then add 1 teaspoon flour, thickened celery stock to cover, and 2 egg yolks mixed with ½ cup light cream. Sprinkle with nutmeg and garnish with sliced truffles.*

With more of an accent on the celery itself, we can recommend the "little celery salad on the side" that appears at many of the best "suppers with covers laid for two," such as the anonymous turn-of-the-century American ditty, "A Midnight Lunch."

*We'll have a little duck, celery salad on the side,*
*A little bottle, cold as ice, in which we may confide....*

*And I will not go home early, for 'tis mean to eat and run:*
*Your Bill of Fare's a dandy, and your Dessert is number one;*

The salad is just the freshest, tenderest mature celery, chopped and seasoned with olive oil, herbed wine vinegar, and a little of the choicest mustard in the house.

## ⸺⟨ EGGPLANT ⟩⸺

In various early English herbals the eggplant is referred to as a "love apple" or "mad apple." Besides showing a common diagnosis of passion as mental illness, these names merely reflect a fear of the vegetable, newly introduced from Spain and Mediterranean Africa, based on its close relationship to henbane and deadly nightshade.

One much distorted Arabian tale attributes aphrodisiac qualities to eggplant baked completely submerged in olive oil, soaking it up like a sponge. The dish supposedly took its name, *imam bayildi* ("fainting priest"), from a holy man's response to an unveiled maiden while eating it. But another, more believable version has the priest marrying a maiden who first cooked the dish for him, then receiving twelve huge jars of olive oil as her dowry. After serving him the eggplant twelve days in a row (some versions say three), the bride did not prepare it on the thirteenth (or fourth). When asked why, she said they were out of olive oil, thus causing the sacerdotal swoon.

The bland, benign, combinable eggplant has almost no nutrients of any kind; its only claim to aphrodisiac fame seems to be in a few recipes where it acts as a vehicle for more stimulating ingredients. An eggplant penis plaster is described on page 203. Following is the dish that reputedly maintained the seminal vigor of the 400-pound Turkish bey Mustafa Mehere through the 170 wives and numberless concubines of his 123-year life (1488–1611). It was concocted by Rada-Hera, the only wife he kept throughout her natural life—apparently because she had the sense to keep her recipe a secret.

*Broil 2 medium eggplants, then peel and purée them. Melt 4 tablespoons butter in a saucepan, add 2 tablespoons flour, and season heavily with white pepper, cayenne, and saffron. Add 1 cup milk, bring to a rapid boil, then simmer, stirring, for 10 minutes. Add ½ cup grated cheese and the juice of ½ lemon, then mix in the eggplant and cook for 5 minutes more before serving.*

## ---◄§ GARLIC AND ONIONS §►---

One day in the early 1920s a Soviet biologist, Alexander Gurvich, made an intriguing discovery. He noticed that his onions were giving off radiation. Specifically, he found that if an onion plant's young growing tip was pointed at the growing tissue of another onion, a dramatic increase in the rate of cell division took place. He named the energy mitogenetic (mitosis-inducing) radiation, M-rays for short. He subsequently found the same emissions coming from garlic and ginseng roots.

Other researchers in Europe duplicated his results, but several scientists in the United States tried and failed. The Academy of Sciences soon concluded Gurvich's work was unreplicable, and M-rays were consigned to limbo as too weird for further research. Now that a later generation of Russians has developed the Kirlian apparatus for photographing auras, there is speculation that M-rays may be a focusing of an organism's energy field, occurring in all growing tissue. There the matter stands, pending further investigation.

Whether or not their effects are due to life-enhancing rays, all these cousins of the lily, the genus *Allium*, have been considered panaceas since prehistoric times. Among humanity's earliest garden crops, onion and garlic were often eaten before war, work, or love to give strength for the task. In fact, the earliest known workers' strike was a walkout of Egyptian pyramid laborers when the garlic supplies ran out. Nearly every herbal ever written recommends the juice or the roasted bulbs to purify the blood, confer vigor, and prevent or treat respiratory infections. Pliny's *Natural History* lists sixty-one diseases susceptible to this magic family.

The legendary Greek aphrodisiac *storgethron* is usually identified by scholars as the leek, and the onion tribe are the vegetables classical men relied upon above all others. A young man, for example, finds himself in a predicament in Aristophanes' *The Women in Politics*. The females have taken over the assembly and decreed a form of communism that tries to eliminate ageism, among other things. A law is passed that would force a man to satisfy an old woman first every time he wants to bed down with a young one. Our hero finds himself nearly torn asunder by two elderly dames who have claimed him at the same moment. When he protests that he can't row two boats at once, he is blamed for not having eaten a hundredweight of onions before leaving his house.

Among the Romans, Martial advised, "If your wife is old and your member is exhausted, eat onions in plenty," and Petronius recommends them as the only accompaniment to a fortifying diet of snails.

When one of the heroes of *The Perfumed Garden*, Abou el-Heïloukh, is required to sustain an erection for thirty days in order to gain the girl of his dreams, he does so merely by drinking onion juice with enough honey to make it palatable. After some experimentation, I would say this is about half and half, or up to two parts of honey to one of juice—if one is willing to expand one's definition of palatable.

Sexologist William J. Robinson added to Allium's anecdotal lore with the results of extensive medical tests in his practice. He emerged convinced that there is "no question as to its *pronounced aphrodisiac effect.* In fact, it stands at the head of the list." He also found that some peoples, notably Italians and Jews, "instinctively" use garlic as a tonic and aphrodisiac in their traditional cuisine, while the Anglo-Saxons and some other northern races would rather be limp than eat it. We can add the French, Arabs, the Caucasus centenarians, and practically all Asians to the list of lusty, long-lived garlic lovers.

Certain lovers of the bulb go so far as to see the entire pageant of human history as a disguised conflict between the forces of alliolatry and alliophobity. Garlic adoration has recently reached new heights with the formation by Lloyd J. Harris of an association called The Lovers of the Stinking Rose (1043 Cragmont Ave., Berkeley, Calif. 94708), and his *The Book of Garlic* and a "digest," *Garlic Times*; the establishment of a restaurant (La Vieille Maison, Truckee, Calif.) so exclusively devoted to garlic that its menu includes garlic ice cream; and the invention of garlic shower therapy by Yoshio Kato and the Oyama Garlic Laboratory in Amagasake, Japan. This is just what it sounds like—an enclosed shower that inundates the patient's every pore with a stimulating, germicidal garlic juice, diluted or full strength.

I am a confirmed alliophile who, in my younger days as a cast-iron gourmet, occasionally got a day off from school by chewing a couple of raw cloves in morning history class, so I'm inclined to believe that where there's smoke there's fire. Science usually confirms, eventually, traditions as universally accepted as the sexual worth of Allium plants. Just why they should be aphrodisiac remains a mystery; but decades of extensive medical tests have proven garlic, and to a lesser extent onions, to be effective in lowering high blood pressure and serum cholesterol levels, promoting healthy digestion, killing a wide variety of unwanted bacteria, clearing up many types of respiratory congestion, and possibly helping the body get rid of poisonous metals like mercury, lead, and cadmium. A compound from onions called allyl-propyl-disulfide (APDS) has been shown to decrease the insulin needs of diabetic rabbits.

Standard nutritional analyses show nothing more interesting in onions than moderately high levels of potassium, while garlic shows a fair amount of potassium, phosphorus, and carbohydrate. Their characteristic odor and flavor is due to several sulfur compounds. Onions contain a tear gas $(CH_3CH_2CH = S = O)$ and APDS $(CH_3CH_2CH_2-S-S-CH_2CH_2 = CH_2)$. Garlic includes the compounds allium $(CH_2 = CHCH_2S-CH_2CHNH_2COOH)$ and allyl sulfide $(CH_2 = CH\ CH_2\ \ S-S-CH_2CH = CH_2)$. Robinson purified this last in the form of "garlic oil," but found it was not as potent as the whole bulb.

There are far too many famous garlic and onion recipes to do justice to them here. There is Spanish *sopa de ajo*, Provençal *aioli* sauce, and chicken with forty cloves. Few modern Western cooks know that onions, like leeks, make a delicious steamed vegetable alone as well as blending well in sauces and sautéed dishes. Fewer still realize that fully cooked garlic becomes an altogether new vegetable—when charcoal-roasted in the skin by the Arabs or cooked in casserole thus:

### ROAST GARLIC
*Place 20 large garlic cloves in a small casserole with 3 tablespoons butter, 1½ tablespoons peanut oil, 1½ tablespoons olive oil, and some salt and pepper. Bake at 350° F. for at least 20 minutes, stirring or basting often. When done they will be soft, starchy, and sweeter than you ever expected.*

You need not worry about losing aphrodisiac nutrients by cooking Alliums; the probable active compounds of sulfur are fairly heat-stable and do not readily dissolve in cooking water. Remember, though, that both partners should share the dish if the postprandial course is to be a success. This is assuming the onions are not being used, as Xenophon suggests, to cover up someone else's perfume.

## ·◄❁ *LEGUMES* ❁►·

Rich in calcium, iron, potassium, and phosphorus, beans are also among the most proteinaceous of vegetables. Combined with other plant proteins or with animal proteins, legumes have been a steady, storable amino acid source through the ages. The soybean, foundation of China, does not even need to be combined with other foods to be an efficient protein source. Whether lima, navy, black, red, broad, haricot, kidney, turtle, hyacinth, or pinto, beans are staples of all farming societies and have warmed us through many a winter. They were thought so generative by the Romans that many took their family names from legumes. The Fabii reckoned their ancestry from the *faba* (bean); the Piso from the *pisa* (pea); the Lentuli from lentils, and the family of Cicero from the Latin for chick-pea.

The concentrated nutrition in beans seems to be the sum total of their aphrodisiac worth, unless we believe the old tale that the gas they produce helps fill out a man's ballooning erection. The oligosaccharides that produce the flatulence, by the way, have recently been bred out of certain experimental strains by U.S. Department of Agriculture scientists.

Ascetics have denounced beans since Pythagoras. Saint Jerome denied beans to the nuns in the fourth-century Jerusalem convent he ran because "they produce titillations in the genital parts"; but the wife of the singer of an old English ballad was much kinder:

*My love hung limp beneath the leaf,*
  *(O bitter, bitter shame!)*
*My heavy heart was full of grief*
  *Until my lady came.*

*She brought a tasty dish to me,*
  *(O swollen pod and springing seed!)*
*My love sprang out right eagerly*
  *To serve me in my need.*

Shaykh Nefzawi recommends the water in which chick-peas were soaked, according to the following formula:

*Heat 1 part onion juice mixed with 2 parts honey "until the onion juice disappears," then dilute the liquid 1:3 with water. Soak chick-peas in this for 24 hours and drink a little of the fluid before bed the next night.*

The confident chieftain predicts that "the member of him who has drunk of it will not give him much rest during the night that follows. . . ." I have noticed no direct effect that I can unhesitatingly ascribe to this procedure. It's possible some of the phosphorus or calcium salts are leached out into the water, but I fail to see why the chick-peas themselves, cooked in some of the liquor, would not be better.

From the *Ananga Ranga* comes a similar recipe. Here it is the seeds of the *uríd* (mung beans) which are soaked, in sugared milk instead of water. The mess is then exposed to the sun for three days (evidently to dry up excess liquid), ground to a powder, kneaded into cakes, and fried in *ghee* (clarified butter). The result would be fairly nutritious, but hardly justifies the assurance that the eater, "though smitten with years . . . will enjoy a hundred women."

Everyone has their own favorite recipe for bean soup, from

the stark ham and beans and water recipe of the official U.S. House of Representatives restaurant, to Boston baked beans (learned from the Indians, who used maple syrup and bear fat instead of molasses and salt pork), to Mexican chili, to Indian dal, to Chinese carp and red bean soup. Here's my preference, from Douglas's *Venus in the Kitchen*:

> *After soaking overnight, cook 1 pound broad beans in salted water with a ham hock or two [try to find hocks smoked without nitrites], a bunch of parsley, and pinch of saffron. Purée most of the beans, save a few whole, and put them all back into just enough of the cooking liquid to make a thick soup. Then add a handful of uncooked rice and perhaps another pinch of saffron and some chopped parsley. Simmer and serve when the rice is done, topped with grated parmesan cheese.*

## ⸙ MUSHROOMS ⸙

Various mushrooms have been named God's flesh in Mexico, the Mediterranean, the Middle East, India, and China, usually because they open the mind's gateway to heaven. Here we are concerned with the less spectacular types that feed the flesh of people. Even these have sometimes been dedicated to gods: food mushrooms among the ancient Greeks were sacred to Eros and the Egyptians reserved mushrooms for the pharaoh-god's table. The phallic glanslike cap and stem of the tender young ones form the signature that proclaimed mushrooms a sex food.

Few details are known about the nutritional value of mushrooms except that they hold moderate amounts of potassium, phosphorus, and niacin. Since they are over 90 percent water, they are not concentrated sources of anything, but they are unique as the only vegetable that contains glycogen. Often called animal starch, glycogen is the form in which our bodies store carbohydrate until it is needed for energy. Mushrooms also produce small amounts of "sunshine" vitamin D, despite their usual habitats of shady woods and dark cellars. When cooked, they act as sponges for oil; in sautéing, 100 grams can increase in caloric content from a mere 7 to a whopping 217. The oil plus the glycogen can help fill the body's energy reserves in the liver and muscles, but no more than many other foods.

There is, at present, no reason to think that food mushrooms contain any aphrodisiac bonus other than what their flavor and shape confer. This is as true of wild varieties as it is of cultivated ones. Furthermore, if you decide to go in search of the exotic tastes of woodland fungi, you must learn the art of collecting from one already experienced in it—not from a guidebook—to avoid a prematurely ended love life. Nor are there any "kitchen tests" to distinguish poisonous from edible; deadly mushrooms will *not* necessarily turn silver black, onions brown, or vinegar cloudy. This consumer problem has so far been solved only in Switzerland, where Geneva's wild-mushroom market offers fifty species, gathered and sold under supervision of a state mycologist.

The edible fungi include certain puffballs, including the giant *Lycoperdon giganteum* or *Calvatia maxima*, sometimes three feet across. The largest are best, having a fragrant flesh a bit like cream cheese. Since they are edible if they grow aboveground and their flesh is white, puffballs are safer to collect, although expert guidance is still a good idea the first time out.

## ---◄{ ROCKET }►---

No one who hasn't tasted the bitterly aromatic yet strangely sweet leaves of the rocket (*rucola* in Italian) can form an adequate idea of their taste. Today arugola is used throughout much of Europe and Italian kitchens in North America. In its Mediterranean homeland, its aphrodisiac renown is voiced by the usual Romans—Ovid, Horace, Martial and Columella—who say it was sacred to Priapus and sown around his ubiquitous phallic statues erected throughout the Roman Empire. They most often ate the young leaves, picked before flowering, in a simple salad as follows:

*Wash and dry a handful of arugola leaves and half a head of lettuce. Dress with olive oil, wine vinegar, salt, pepper, and a clove of minced garlic.*

Nutritional information on rocket is hard to come by, but ancient and Renaissance doctors regularly recommended it for diseases of the lungs and urinary tract. Today, because of a high vitamin C content, it is considered mainly an antiscorbutic. Once placed in the cabbage family as *Brassica eruca,* dame's or garden, white or purple, rocket is today usually given a genus of its own, *Eruca sativa.*

Arugola makes a tasty salad but is hardly a sure-fire love food, especially if both parties don't agree on the taste. Who knows whether ancient varieties contained something the modern ones do not, or if perhaps the aromatic oils do have some cumulative effect. Perhaps rocket's fame comes partly from its significance as the flower of deceit—Hesperis or vesper flower—for its orange-scented blossoms give a delicious perfume by evening but none during the day.

No matter why, I love it and believe in it. I compete with Italian restaurants for the neighborhood supply. And when there is none available, I make do with a similarly piquant green—fresh coriander tops, also called Chinese parsley and *cilantro.*

## ⊶ TRUFFLES ⊷

For centuries an untold number of men and women have tried to pin down in words the flavor and aroma of the truffle. An equal number have devised various means of hunting them, often in cooperation with animals. Others have tried to tame them for cultivation like other food crops. After all these efforts, the truffle remains today the most elusive vegetable. Constant throughout its history have been its rarity and aphrodisiac fame.

The truffle is a fungus, anywhere from a nut to a melon in size, that grows a few inches to a few feet underground in a symbiotic relationship with the roots of trees, usually oak or beech. They are gathered commercially in southern France and northern Italy.

In France the centers of production are in the districts of Quercy-Périgord, east of Bordeaux, and Vaucluse-Gard, north of Marseilles. Here grows *Tuber melanosporum*, whose brown or violet-tinged black flesh with its gray marbling is so desired that, even where they are most plentiful, black truffles are locked in restaurant safes.

They are dug late in autumn, some being shipped fresh to the United States as late as January or February. The crop varies with the weather from year to year; when there is enough rain to produce a bad vintage, there is enough for an excellent truffle harvest. About a quarter of the take is exported, but the estimated total varies widely from source to source—anywhere from a hundred to a thousand tons per year.

In the Umbrian district of Italy, northeast of Rome, and near Alba in the Piedmont, lurks *Tuber magnatum*, the summer or white truffle, in contrast to the French variety, even though "white" is really brown or beige. It is rarer than the black and often considered less tasty, although many prefer its hint of garlic to the more peppery *melanosporum*. The land on which it grows, and thus the supply, is controlled almost exclusively by two families, the Morras and the Urbanis, who do business in a rivalry as intense as that between the Hatfields and McCoys.

In both regions the tubers are sometimes sought by skilled gatherers who can spot those near the surface when they crack the ground or starve the grass. Some can find them by smell, and divining rods have even been tried in Greece. Most *caveurs* (truffle hunters), however, work with an animal of some kind. In France the favorites are pigs, especially young sows, who are trundled to the truffle ground in a wheelbarrow. Then, on a leash, they are allowed to root up the tuber, but pulled back before they can eat it.

In Italy poodles, hounds, dachshunds, or terriers are preferred, but since dogs do not naturally eat truffles, they must be taught the trade, often in the Monchiero truffle-dog school in Alba. Those who prefer pigs claim dogs have inferior truffle noses and stray after game, while dog users say pigs tire too fast and are not obedient. Some gatherers simply prefer to watch the ground for the truffle flies that eat the fungi, lay eggs on them, and help spread the truffle spores.

Truffles do flourish elsewhere, but the quality usually does not approach the French and Italian types. Local varieties are sometimes sold in England. The Russians have tried to solve the pig-dog controversy by harvesting theirs with bear cubs; the Sardinians, with goats. At least forty species grow in the United States (some have even been found in New York's Central Park), but they are too rare and unappetizing to bother with. The best non-European ones grow in southern Africa, where !Kung bushmen eat huge amounts of them for dessert—after their staples of snake, lizard, and grubs. Western buyers are eager, but the !Kung love them and are reluctant to sell.

In his *Memorials of Gourmandising*, William Makepeace Thackeray wrote that the truffles were announced by their odor— "musky, fiery, savory, mysterious—a hot drowsy smell, that lulls the senses, and yet enflames them. . . ." This bouquet, sometimes likened to filberts and cheese, is so powerful that truffles may be used twice. If left refrigerated overnight with broken eggs, then removed, they can flavor scrambled eggs at breakfast and still garnish a soup for lunch.

Both Italian and French varieties are available canned throughout the United States at an average price of twelve to fifteen dollars an ounce. This form is better than nothing, but still only a pale shadow of the pungent fresh ones. When added to dishes, they should be merely heated, not cooked, so as to retain what savor they have left.

The diamond of cookery is best appreciated when freshly unearthed, well cut, and mounted in a simple but elegant setting. The tough, warty rind should be well scrubbed. For most purposes they are sliced paper-thin or grated for maximum aroma. Given their rarity and renown, the amount of culinary invention lavished on them is hardly surprising. The best single source of truffle recipes is probably Charles Heartman's *Cuisine de l'amour*. From this collection comes a Russian salad by way of Alexandre Dumas (père):

> *Peel some black truffles and cook them for 3 or 4 minutes in a casserole with a little Madeira and salt. Slice thinly into an earthen pot and let them stand with a little oil for 10 minutes. Sprinkle them with tarragon, chives, and chopped parsley, and mix with a bit of fresh mayonnaise. Serve on a platter topped with more mayonnaise and a spoonful of English mustard.*

They can be puréed:

> *Have a béchamel sauce ready. Grate the truffles and add them to the sauce with a glass of sherry and 1 teaspoon heavy cream. Heat gently, do not boil.*

The Romans, who imported some from Greece but especially loved the reddish ones from Libya, favored this recipe recorded by Apicius:

> *Slice the truffles to a moderate thickness, sprinkle with salt, and simmer in water very briefly, then spear them on twigs and roast over a fire till partly done. Beat some flour into a mixture of oil, wine, honey, and pepper as it*

*heats in a saucepan; finish the truffles in this liquid, and eat from the twigs.*

If you ever find yourself able to afford a meal of several whole ones the size of potatoes, you might try this:

*Wrap each truffle in 5 or 6 sheets of heavy paper soaked in water, then roast in hot coals. If desired, they may be sprinkled with cognac and wrapped in salt pork with less paper. Watch their progress carefully; when done, remove paper, wipe away any ashes, and serve on a silver tray. (If you can afford the tubers, the tray should be no problem.)*

Scores of other time-tested recipes could be added. Rabelais's favorite snack of oysters with truffled sausages could be reconstructed. Wealthy readers could dine on the turkey completely stuffed with truffles that was so popular during the French aristocracy's pre-Revolutionary era of gastronomic potlatch. There are Alice B. Toklas's truffle turnovers and the truffled vanilla ice cream created by Lorenzo Delmonico for a millionaire's dinner competition in New York's Gay Nineties.

But are truffles really an aphrodisiac? Malençon's authoritative monograph of 1938 ("European Truffles: History, Morphogenesis, Organography, Classification, Culture") does not answer it. They are absent from most nutritional texts, but Dr. Arnold Lorand postulated they are good sources of phosphorus and iron. That alone would make them no more potent than halibut and parsley, however.

Of the two occasions I have been able to sample this delicacy, once I had no opportunity for lovemaking afterward, and the other time I did so more out of a sense of expectation than from any perceptible result of the meal. Hence, I would not take my own word on this matter.

In his attempt to find the answer, Brillat-Savarin interviewed many gourmets and for the most part got only sly, evasive answers. But from one elderly and unaffected woman he heard this tale: When much younger the lady once dined with her husband and a good friend (male) on a magnificent truffled fowl. Soon after dessert her husband had to leave for a business appointment. As the evening passed, their friend grew affable, then expansive, then complimentary, then persuasive, and finally so energetically demonstrative that even the dazed wife could not mistake the gleam in his eye. With the utmost difficulty she marshaled her reserves of honor against the promptings of her own body and her friend's, and escaped with a false promise of "some other time." Afterward, she unhesitatingly blamed the near faux pas on the truffles.

Who can tell, in a specific case, whether such inopportune desire really comes from the entrée? The professor of gastronomy at length concluded: "The truffle is not a positive aphrodisiac; but it can, in certain situations, make women tenderer and men more agreeable." French chef Jacques Manière has said a pound per day would make a man one of the world's greatest lovers.

Even the poor may soon be able to put this claim to the test, if recent news from France is correct. A team of agronomists say they have harvested twenty truffles from a bed they seeded three and a half years earlier. If so, the truffle, which has foiled all previous attempts at cultivation, may at last be domesticated. Since a truffle bed doesn't reach commercial potential for at least five years after its inception, and needs twenty to forty years to reach its peak, we will not know the full results for some time. If it turns out that truffles can be grown in low-priced quantity like any other fungus, it will be interesting to see whether their reputed aphrodisiac powers wane.

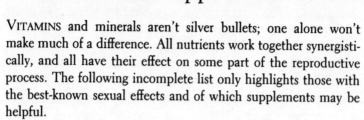

# Vitamin and Mineral Supplements

VITAMINS and minerals aren't silver bullets; one alone won't make much of a difference. All nutrients work together synergistically, and all have their effect on some part of the reproductive process. The following incomplete list only highlights those with the best-known sexual effects and of which supplements may be helpful.

)»— *Vitamin A*  Besides being needed for proper vision, vitamin A is essential in some as yet unknown way for the health of the skin and mucous membranes, and the production of all sex hormones. For this reason a daily dose of cod liver oil has sometimes been found to improve sexual function. Care must be taken in supplementing vitamin A, since it is stored in the liver and becomes toxic in excess. Total daily intake of A (from food and supplements) should not exceed 50,000 units for long periods of time.

)»— *B complex vitamins*  No one knows how many B vitamins there are—probably about two dozen. They are essential to the burning of food for energy and to most other processes of every cell in the body.

Like most of the B complex, *pantothenic acid* is vital to hormone formation. Humans are especially prone to a pantothenic deficiency because we have a higher tissue level of it than most of the foods we eat, so it is often a good choice for supplementation.

None of the B complex vitamins can be disregarded. A pyridoxine ($B_6$) deficiency can cause impotence in men. A lack of thiamine ($B_1$), riboflavin ($B_2$), or choline can upset the liver's regulation of the relative amounts of the testosterone and estrogen circulating in each of us. If too much estrogen accumulates in a male, for example, sterility can result.

Some users of the newly marketed *pangamic acid* or *calcium pangamate* ($B_{15}$) have reported an astounding surge of erotic interest, as well as longer, more intense orgasms. First found in apricot pits by laetrile discoverer E. T. Krebs in 1951, $B_{15}$ is not officially a vitamin because no deficiency disease has been found for it. The Food and Drug Administration allows its marketing for lack of a reason to ban it.

Russian doctors claim miraculous $B_{15}$ benefits for their heart patients. Scores of Soviet research papers maintain that it raises energy by improving oxygen transport to the cells and that it aids protein synthesis and helps regulate steroid hormone levels. And it's selling like hot *blini*. Dr. Yakov Shpirt of Moscow Clinical Hospital No. 60 recommends it with the advice, "We must not fear universal remedies."

Back in the U.S.A., Muhammad Ali, overweight and lackadaisical while training for the Jimmy Young fight in 1976, turned the corner when he started taking $B_{15}$ and other supplements suggested by Dr. Richard Passwater. If writing a book is anything like prizefighting, I can credit $B_{15}$ with the last-minute lift needed to complete the final pages of the present volume. $B_{15}$ has quickly moved from an exotic performance supplement for athletes to the hottest health food since vitamin E, even at $8 for 100 50-milligram tablets. Daily doses are usually 50–150 milligrams.

*Vitamin C*  A full list of all the body's uses for ascorbic acid would fill a small encyclopedia. Its indirect sexual effects are basically three: it is essential for healthy collagen, the "intercellular cement" that holds all our cells solidly together—it keeps us tight; it assists proper cell oxygenation; and it is crucial to proper function of the adrenal glands—thus it is another antifatigue factor.

The U.S. recommended daily allowance of 35–60 milligrams is enough to prevent scurvy, but not much else. Vitamin C researchers suggest 500–3,000 milligrams daily for optimum health (more during illness or stress), preferably divided into three doses taken before meals.

*Vitamin D*   Calcium and phosphorus cannot be absorbed in the intestine without vitamin D, which is best known for building these minerals into bones and teeth. But phosphorus would also be unavailable for sex hormones without D. An oil-soluble vitamin, D is more dangerous than A. It is unwise to add more than 1,000 units to the daily diet, and total intakes over 1,800 units can cause nausea, diarrhea, vomiting, weight loss, and bed-wetting. Anyone who gets a lot of unpolluted sunshine should not need extra D.

*Vitamin E*   The oil-soluble tocopherol compounds collectively called vitamin E have been overrated as the "sex vitamin" ever since their discoverers in the 1920s found that a deficiency causes sterility in rats. Vitamin E is essential to gonadic function, but no more so than many other nutrients. It functions as an antioxidant to protect hormones and cell walls from deterioration. It can also increase stamina somewhat by promoting more efficient use of oxygen in the body. It has been found helpful in some cases of sterility in both sexes and helps prevent perinatal complications in pregnancy. It is especially concentrated in the anterior pituitary, which regulates the synthesis of sex hormones.

The best natural sources of vitamin E are wheat germ oil, other *unheated* vegetable oils, nuts and seeds, eggs, leafy green vegetables, and meat, especially rabbit and steak tartare. Persons with diabetes, high blood pressure, heart damage, or thyroid problems should take vitamin E supplements only under the guidance of a doctor, as disturbing side effects can appear from suddenly increased intake. For most people, amounts of 100–800 units daily are harmless and may provide noticeable benefits. The vitamin is best absorbed when taken after a meal containing oil or fat.

☙— *Phosphorus* This element was probably the first mineral found to be directly linked to sexual arousal. Horniness was and still is an occupational hazard of phosphorus refiners. John Davenport, in the first full-length study of aphrodisiacs in English, tells the tale of a pharmacist's pet drake who drank water out of a vessel in which phosphorus had previously been kept and "ceased not gallanting his females till he died." Many old recipes survive for the use of pure phosphorus, but it's too easy to overdose oneself to death this way. It is much better to get one's supply from organic sources, the richest of which are fish, eggs, milk, nuts, seeds, and beans. I wish to testify that a diet of fish once or twice a day tends to become very interesting toward the end of the first week. Phosphorus is an integral part of many sex hormones; in balance with calcium, it builds bones and enables nerves and brain to function—hence the additional reputation of fish as mind food.

☙— *Zinc* This mineral has only been recognized as an essential nutrient for a decade or so. Both sexes make hormones with zinc, but it's especially important for sperm and seminal fluid. Deficiencies, common because most soils today lack zinc, can cause retarded sexual development in adolescents and prostatitis in older men. Its best natural sources are oysters, other seafood, milk, pumpkin and sunflower seeds, wheat bran and germ, and oatmeal. The amount needed daily is about 15 milligrams. Supplementation sounds like a good idea for women and more so for men who have an active sex life and/or a diet low in natural sources. Noting that zinc loss in extended intercourse could add up to 2 or more milligrams, Dr. Carl Pfeiffer reluctantly conceded there may have been a grain of truth in the old scarums about masturbation leading to insanity. Ejaculatory loss in an already zinc-deficient male could lead to serious depletion of the areas of the brain richest in zinc—the pineal body, which apparently regulates sexual cycles, and the hippocampus, which mediates emotions.

*Iodine* This is another mineral that may be deficient in people who eat little seafood. An adequate supply is essential for the thyroid gland to regulate the metabolic rate and energy level. An underactive thyroid usually means little interest in sex, as well as other aspects of life. Iodized salt is one source, but it may mean getting too much salt to get enough iodine. The best organic source is kelp. This is a general name for any of the edible brown, green, blue, or red sea algae, commonly used as food in Ireland and the Orient. Besides giving us iodine, they help return to our diet trace minerals that are constantly being washed by rain out of the soil into the sea.

*Manganese* About 4 milligrams of this metal are needed daily to form nucleic acids and other proteins. It is also used for thyroxine and the enzymes that control glandular secretions activating the maternal instinct.

*Selenium* Supplements of this mineral are routinely given to farm animals to ensure normal reproduction, but its effects in humans are little tested. Selenium-deficient male rats are often sterile, forming few sperm cells, with poor motility due to flagella that break off. Selenium concentrates in the gonads of both sexes, but less in women than men. Selenium may contribute to baby survival; infant death rates are statistically higher in areas where soils lack it. Controlled human tests are absent, but some men and women who have taken supplements (usually 150–200 *mi-crograms* daily) have noted dramatic "desire swells."

}⟡— *Vanadium*   This little-known element seems to be an essential trace mineral in humans, because it is found in most tissues, rapidly excreted, and shows no known toxicity even in high doses. Vanadium deficiency has been shown to slow the reproductive rate of rats. Our main sources are corn, soy, and olive oils and black pepper. It is also produced by burning coal and oil—the only known beneficial component of air pollution.

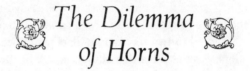

# The Dilemma of Horns

A SMALL ungulate called McNeill's deer, native to the Tibetan plateau, is nearly extinct today because its antler velvet is much in demand as an aphrodisiac on the Asian market. The musk deer is also rare and declining because its gential secretions smell so good to humans. As of 1977, we were down to the last fifty Javan rhinoceroses. The East African square-lipped or white rhino and the Sumatran rhino have fared a little better; in 1977 there were just over a hundred of each in the wild. Of rhinos, only the black variety is not an immediately endangered species. Other animals have been decimated by hunting or simple human expansion into the wilds, but the species mentioned here are primarily victims of the lust for elixirs.

Even our ancestors are not exempt. In 1927 an incomplete skull of Peking man was found—the largest relic of this Pleistocene predecessor then known. Two years later, as the Japanese prepared their invasion, the skull was packed for safe transport out of the country. But when the crate reached Shanghai, its keepers found *they* had been shanghaied. The skull had been stolen and probably ground to powder for the "aphrodisiac" fossil trade then flourishing in China.

There is no way to tell how this faith in horn and old bone arose, except to point the finger of symbolism. For the record, rhino horn is composed of keratin (the tough protein that forms most animal horns and hooves), thiolactic acid (lactic acid with a bivalent sulfur replacing an oxygen), two nonessential amino acids (tyrosine and cystine), and two commonly found minerals, calcium carbonate and calcium phosphate.

There seems to be no material reason for any animal prong's lascivious fame, except for a bit of phosphate as easily supplied by fish. Still, the limited supply of rhino horn continues to go at auction for five hundred to two thousand dollars per ounce. It is just as much a fantasy as the belief that all poisons are neutralized in a rhino-horn cup, an idea that made the horn indispensable in every palace and pharmacy of Europe through the seventeenth century. From Dublin to Tokyo, rhino skin and toenails in an oil solution, as well as the horn, were used for innumerable ailments, and toothaches were cured by smoking through cigarette holders made from rhino ribs. Today for three hundred dollars it is still possible to get dinner with a sprinkling of rhino powder on the entrée in Tokyo, Hong Kong, and Singapore.

Oddly enough, although the Chinese and other cultures use hartshorn and dinosaur fossils as sexual tonics, most doctors of traditional Chinese medicine don't recognize any erotic value of rhino horn. They use it only as a sedative and cardiotonic, as they would any source of calcium. But the point is not whether the animal horns work. The point is that, somewhere between the Stone Age hunter's diligent use of every part of the kill and the modern hunter's mechanized slaughter for the apothecary's bottle, something went very wrong. The question is whether there is time to mend it.

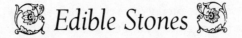 *Edible Stones*

*Is there a man among you who will offer
his son a stone when he asks for bread? . . .*
—JESUS, from "The Sermon
on the Mount"

THE fascinating dazzle and smoothness of gemstones make them
an ideal focus for the psychic energies of their holders and behold-
ers, so it is no wonder that some—notably diamond, sapphire, am-
ethyst, garnet, agate, and aquamarine—have been prized as love
talismans. In fact there is something about any kind of rock—originally congealed fire from the center of the earth—that suggests
the flame that keeps the concealed spark of life burning from generation to generation. Rock, the most plentiful solid of the three
states of matter, shows the sexual attraction (cohesion) of atoms
in the most intense degree.

Most pertinent to our search are the stones that are eaten. Ingestible rocks are generally thought to be aphrodisiacs. Otherwise,
why bother with such fare? And because they are so rare, stones
made by animals are invested with more sexual magic than others.
Pearls, which had the likeness of the lunar fertility goddess going
for them, were sought to keep or restore vigor. Fortunes of them
were stirred into wine or vinegar as an elixir of wealthy lust. The
most famous was probably the 74-carat earring, worth 6 million
sesterces (about $750,000), which Cleopatra gave Antony to
drink with the words, "Don't worry, the dinner cost much more
than that." Pearls *will* dissolve in weak acids if first crushed, being
91.7 percent calcium carbonate. The association of oyster stones
with moon babies is taught by an ancient sacrifice that may still
be done among the pearl fishers of Borneo: Every ninth (a universally sacred number) pearl was stoppered in a bottle with two

grains of rice and a dead man's finger until it "reproduced"—led the diver to more mollusk baubles.

Other creatures produced even more marvelous gems. The wild goat or bezoar antelope of Persia (as well as other ruminants) occasionally contained a similar layered concretion around an irritant, such as a partly digested hairball in its stomach. This bezoar stone was worth a king's ransom as a universal antidote to poisons and a preserver of youth.

In 1978, Andrew A. Benson of the Scripps Institute of Oceanography in San Diego discovered that bezoar stones work, at least for arsenic. Dr. Benson, while investigating the death of algae from industrial pollution in the Pacific, found certain tropical algae with the ability to absorb arsenic and store it in a chemically combined form that is harmless to them. Bezoar stones, Benson found, absorb and combine with arsenic in the same way. This discovery hints of no aphrodisiacal use, but animal stones are still being sold as such. In Brisbane, Australia, the Queensland Chemical Company sells powdered cows' gallstones at sixty-nine dollars an ounce. The company reportedly cannot keep up with local demand, but is considering export.

Likewise the allectorius, once in a blue moon found in the liver of an aged capon, was an infallible attractant that assured its owner the love of whomever he or she desired. Was not its very name, from the Latin verb "to allure," derived from Allecto, the irresistible member of the three Furies?

Others sought to get their rocks off with the aid of pebbles found in the heads of toads, the balance stones in the heads of perch, or the seal of the snake, sought by Muslims in snakes' heads. Albertus Magnus, that thirteenth-century proto-empiricist theologian, recommends the eaglestone—alias *aetites, echites,* or *aquileus*—so-called because eagles were said to seek it for decorating their nests, making its acquisition most difficult. The names refer to a hollow geode, with one or more pebbles inside, causing it to rattle when shaken. Any stone with another stone inside it would naturally evoke associations with eggs and reproduction, so the eaglestone was thought to engender conjugal love when worn from the left shoulder, and also to ensure an easy and normal birth when worn by a pregnant woman.

The mere identity of some of these nuggets will forever remain a mystery. Pliny the Elder briefly mentions a certain "red on white" aphrodisiac stone in his *Natural History,* but rather prudishly withholds its name. Metrodorus, a disciple of the philosopher Epicurus, mentions one called *paneros* ("all-sex"), but neglects details.

Fortunately for us, rocks do not always just lie there waiting to be made into obelisks. They are constantly being worn away to form soil, they dissolve in water, they permeate the sap of plants and our own blood, and they resolidify as bones. Even in solution they may sometimes excite human passion; they would be especially likely to do this, for example, in areas where zinc was unusually abundant. Whether this has ever occurred would be hard to prove, but there are stories of the waters of certain areas having noticeable erotic effects.

In the form of soil, rocks also have erotic effects on humans. This is not to speak of crop fecundity, but rather of pica or geophagy—literally, rock eating. This craving shows up in cases of mineral deficiency due to malnutrition and is most common during pregnancy. As such it frequently occurs among the poor of the rural South, where it may involve eating chalk or laundry starch. Duke University doctors who have studied it found people whose clay habits were up to 4.5 ounces a day and found it nearly impossible to give up, despite severe constipation. Nevertheless, geophagy is sometimes practiced by people whose diet is adequate and who, in effect, choose to eat dirt. Geophagy occurs all over the world, and the best dirt is always considered kaolin, a fine, whitish clay composed of oxides of aluminum and silicon. Although Kaopectate may not seem like much of an aphrodisiac, geophagists generally seem to associate their hobby with a special feeling of erotic well-being; many are known to walk long distances when they find a clay that increases their sexual capacity. They have been described plunging headfirst into an especially good vein, while a friend waits nearby to pull them out when a wiggle of their toes signals they have finished their meal.

The explorer Baron Alexander von Humboldt described the Ottomaques of the Orinoco as eating up to a pound a day of a "fat, unctuous" kaolin tinged with iron oxide which they shape into spheres, bake by a slow fire, and stack by their huts like cannonballs. The Quechua of Peru used to soak their potatoes in a clay and water mixture. A *bergmehl* ("mountain meal") of clay and water is still known in Sweden, as is bread spread with "stone butter" near Germany's Kiffhausen quarries. The natives of Aleppo once reserved an especially fine fuller's earth, *byloon*, for their pregnant women, and *ampo*, a red clay, was eaten in Java for added bodily grace and attractiveness.

Despite the venerable history of geologic love potions, I have not been persuaded to try a side dish of loam, and I would not eat a pearl if I had one. Still, I wonder if M. Lotito ("Mange-tout") is erotically energized by the bicycles and television sets that he eats in two or three weeks as promotional stunts for fairs and charities.

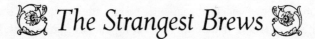 *The Strangest Brews*

ALL'S fair in love and war, we are told, but even the foulest K rations cannot match some of the things that have been swallowed in the name of love. Let's throw some light on the dark corners of our medicine cabinet.

Some of the bottles are empty. Fantastical mixtures like the one Volpone offered Celia—"The milk of unicorns, and panthers' breath/ Gathered in bags ..."—do not age well. Most of the others smell bad.

The Shaykh Nefzawi suggests rubbing the penis with jackal urine to increase its vigor. Many of our medicines list human or animal urine on the label for internal use. One from China is powdered Venus's-comb shell soaked for three days in urine, sun-dried, steeped in donkey water for three days and dried, then sprinkled with flower nectar to kill the taste. Urolagniacs will be glad to know that the urine of healthy males contains a small amount of testosterone. Hormone traces are also found in women's urine and menstrual blood.

The seventeenth-century countess Elizabeth Bathory thought blood was rejuvenating, but she required large amounts of it. She felt an occasional bath in the stuff got her aging juices flowing the way a drink did Dracula's. She drained more than eighty peasant girls from her estate to draw her baths before she was convicted and imprisoned for the rest of her reborn life.

Minski, the anthropophagous giant who appears in most of the Marquis de Sade's novels, credited his ten-times-a-night at the age of forty-five to his dietary supplement of human flesh. A certain number of people in the real world were inclined to agree with him that, once the initial repugnance is overcome, no other food compares with the strength and vigor the flesh of our neighbor imparts, and one can never get enough. Although it is unlikely to be experimentally tested, a case can be made for a direct transfer of metabolic energy that could not happen between organisms of different species. It may have been this thought that led to the adoption of controlled (and sometimes uncontrolled) cannibalism, usually in the form of ritual sacrifice, in so many ancient societies. Peoples as far apart as Ireland and New Guinea once ate the bodies of those who had died a natural death, and, no matter how the death occurred, the eaten were venerated or placated by rite. There is thus more than perversity in the witch's love potion quoted by Horace—human liver and marrow.

The life of a fifteenth-century Scottish cannibal, Sawney Beane, is an advertisement for this aphrodisiac. Beane produced fourteen children and thirty-two grandchildren who hunted as a pack and had more than a thousand wayfarers "for dinner" in a twenty-five-year reign at a stronghold on the Galloway coast.

The human element was retained in many of the medieval and Renaissance philters whose recipes survive, often with the added provision that the flesh must be putrefied. Remember that medieval worship of authority and need for fantasy gave rise to the curious literature known as Books of Secrets. The most famous is the one attributed to Albertus Magnus. He was himself interested in magic, but the book attributed to him is spurious except for the part on stones and a few other chapters, as were similar collections written under the names of Aristotle, Plato, and Galen. They illustrate sympathetic magic in its most gullible form, and it is impossible to tell how much they reflect the actual practices of witches and how much society's lurid dreams about them. Some belief adhered to them in earlier years, but by the sixteenth century they had become mainly light reading for the new public generated by the printing press.

From that period comes a typical hogo quoted in Girolamo Folengo's *Maccaronea** of 1519: "Dry and mix together black dust from a tomb, venom of a toad, flesh of an executed brigand, lung of an ass, blood of a *blind* baby, bile of an ox, and flesh of an exhumed corpse." [Italics added]

But the Renaissance penchant for trying all possible permu-

---

* Girolamo Folengo (1491?–1544), one of Italy's funniest poets, developed the student game of macaronic verse—which slides giddily between classroom Latin and barroom Italian—into a sharp tool for satire. He was given the name Teofilo when, following family tradition, he became a Benedictine monk in 1509. His masterfully sinful epic, *Baldus*, appeared in 1517 under the name Merlin Cocai. After greatly adding to a revised edition (1521), which influenced Rabelais, Folengo gained release from his vows and wrote more macaronics, notably "The Chaos of a Three-Part Man." Finally undergoing a three-year hermitage to reenter monkhood, he (as Teofilo) atoned with some dull holy verse and the appropriately titled *Janus*, an apology for his former scurrility. In secret, however, he still sauced his macaronics; the last edition of *Baldus* emerged posthumously in 1552 from the notes he had left his brother Giambattista, also a monk.

tations of common and rare material, in hopes they would suddenly fuse into a dimly envisioned panacea, is best visible by the light of satire, from the mouth of Pertinax Surly in Jonson's *The Alchemist*, laughing at all the contradictory brews:

> [*What else than card tricks are*]
> . . . *your elixir, your* lac virginis,
> *Your stone, your med'cine, and your chrysosperme,*
> *Your sal, your sulphur, and your mercury,*
> *Your oil of height, your tree of life, your blood,*
> *Your marchesite, your tutie, your magnesia,*
> *Your toad, your crow, your dragon, and your panther;*
> *Your sun, your moon, your firmament, your adrop,*
> *Your lato, azoch, zernich, chilbrit, heautarit,*
> *And then your red man, and your white woman,*
> *With all your broths, your menstrues, and materials*
> *Of piss and egg-shells, women's terms, man's blood,*
> *Hair o' the head, burnt clouts, chalk, merds, and clay,*
> *Powder of bones, scalings of iron, glass,*
> *And worlds of other strange ingredients,*
> *Would burst a man to name?*

But even this powerful stew has to give way to the macho simplicity of our first runner-up, from the Old West: a double of rum and a spoon of black gunpowder in a mug of hot water. And from the far-out East of Sikkim comes the Zen purity of the grand champion: a cup of water in which the rare Himalayan *ken fo* bird has shat.

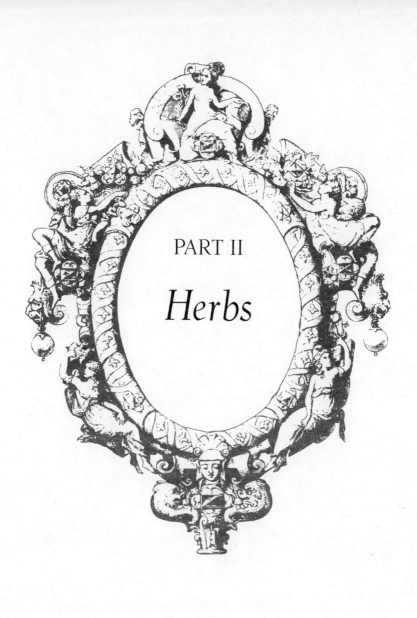

PART II

*Herbs*

*I am not as was Hercules the stout,*
*That to the seventh journey could hold out;*
*I want those herbs and roots of Indian soil,*
*That strengthen weary members in their toil*
*Or drugs or electuaries of new devises,*
*That shame my purse, and tremble at the prices.*
　　　　　—THOMAS NASH, c. 1601, from
　　　　"The Merie Ballad of Nash, His Dildo"

THE noble and ill-rewarded quest for aphrodisiac plants has no
known beginning. It may have been part of our most ancient
herbal lore, the instinctive knowledge of healing leaves carried
over from our tree-dwelling primate past. Two separate traditions
seem to have developed—one group of herbs to promote the
woman's fertility, the tribe's future, and another to raise the man
in her estimation. The search for the male aphrodisiac has been
more prominent, or at least better publicized, in our five thousand
years of history, all written after the discovery of the father's role
in conception.

Our earliest historical records show the use of aphrodisiacs already firmly established. The Egyptians sent their mummified pharaohs erect to their final rest with jars of spice and pepper. The dangers were well known to Augustan Rome, a society that used so many love potions that crowds at vendors' stalls blocked traffic in their sector of the Forum. Next to prostitution, the herb and amulet trade was probably the biggest business in the Subura, the Times Square of Rome between the Esquiline and Viminal hills. The poet Lucretius was, according to Eusebius Pamphili, driven mad by a potion given him by his wife. He managed to write a bit more in intervals of lucidity, but finally killed himself at the age of forty-four. Finally, the Lex Cornelia under Vespasian decreed a fine and deportation for aphrodisiac vendors and death for murder if their concoctions killed.

Other herbs were known to bring energy or euphoria or otherwise tickle the urge indirectly, but by and large the pagan world held the true aphrodisiac to be a mirage, although worth looking for, just in case. But until the fifteenth century, much of medieval Europe believed in the sure-shot potion with the same faith bestowed on the Holy Grail. If it could not be found between the lines of Aristotle or Galen, then surely it would one day turn up among the endless variations of ritual spells or toad-heart-root-and-dung mixtures which, as Books of Secrets, became the comic books of Elizabethan England.

During the age of the great herbals, in the sixteenth and seventeenth centuries, doctors and botanists took a fresh look at herbs, reviving ancient empiricism and laying the foundations of modern medicine and botany. The search for magic potions like *aurum potabile* ("drinkable gold") continued, but there was new emphasis on the gradual tonic properties of plants used daily for weeks or months. There was particular interest in diuretics and digestive tonics, due to a diet high in meat and starch, especially among the upper classes.

The age of exploration brought hundreds of new plants and many exotic aphrodisiacs back to Europe. This process continues in ethnobotany today. But for the most part the decline of the herbals signaled a change in the quest. Medicine packed its bag with purified drugs, ever more powerful, and plants were relegated to colors in a vase or wallpaper. The age most obsessed with aphrodisiacs, the eighteenth century, saw the vogue of phosphorus and cantharides, later followed by arsenic and strychnine.

This era also saw the rebirth of the pill-and-lotion industry, heralded by such brands as Electuaire Satyrion. The trade fit right in with the patent-medicine boom of the nineteenth century. When Anthony Comstock, perhaps the J. Edgar Hoover of sex, got a law passed in his name in 1873 outlawing "obscene" material in the mails, his office (of course he was made commissioner) seized thirty thousand boxes of aphrodisiacs in its first year—along with sixty thousand condoms and five thousand decks of cards.

Dr. Magnus Hirschfeld wrote that "out of a hundred sexual stimulants, one perhaps is efficacious; but ninety of them are an excellent business proposition." Today this is untrue; the market is small and overcrowded, though very steady. Effective stimulants are mostly either illegal, fattening, or sold by prescription only; interest in the others seems limited mostly to the poor and the desperate.

In the 1970s a growing market for legal herbal highs has been generated as a spin-off from the enormous market for illegal highs. Among its best sellers are herbs with some aphrodisiac pretensions. Mail order companies like Woodley Herber, Herbal Holding Company, Home Grown Herbs, and many others sell effective mixtures of yohimbé, damiana, hops, kavakava, muira puama, et cetera. Some companies sell guarana as an aphrodisiac, trading on its exotic name and South American origin, even though the seeds of this woody vine are stimulating only by virtue of their high concentration of caffeine.

Health food stores carry many of the herbs discussed here, such as ginseng, gotu kola, licorice, and sarsaparilla. Many cities have herb shops that can supply most of them. You will probably have to go to a Chinese pharmacy for fleeceflower root and to an Indian grocery for asafetida and (if you're lucky) betel nuts. Dita seeds and burra gokhru are almost impossible to find in the United States. A partial list of major herb suppliers may be found in the Appendix on page 223. When experimenting, please heed one word of caution: When trying any unfamiliar herb or drug, it is a good idea to start with *half* of the suggested *minimum* dose and gradually work upwards, because individuals vary widely in their sensitivity.

Other herbs will surely enter the trade as ethnopharmacologists try out the obscure aphrodisiacs still used by the uncivilized, such as:

)%--- The juice of *ric* leaves (a plant of the lily family), used to promote erections in the Caroline Islands

)%--- Peruvian *huanarpo macho* (*Jatropha angusta*), which abets desire in opposition to the "female" form of the plant

)%--- The *vilca* seeds (*Anadenanthera colubrina*) of the Bolivian Callahuayos, boiled in water, with honey

)%--- Mexican *cundeamor*, or "love spreader" (*Momordica charantia*), related to wild cucumber

)%--- The oval, bittersweet seeds of the Malay scurf pea, called *P'o ku chi* in China and *babchi* in India, containing the alkaloid psoralein or poraline and used for impotence

)%--- *Yin yang ts'ao* (*Epimedium macranthum*), a Chinese restorative of potency and fertility

⟩⟩— *Malabaila sekakul* of the North African Arabs

⟩⟩— Sudanese *Cussonia nigerica*, which dries up excess vaginal juices while aiding the flow of lust

⟩⟩— Southern Asia's bastard teak (*Butea monosperma*)

⟩⟩— The Zambian confetti tree root (*Maytenus senegalensis*), which the natives whittle into their beer

Despite the influx of new herbs, the mainstream of the industry, advertised between the life-size pump-up go-go dolls and the x-ray sin glasses ("Get a Broad View of the World") in the back pages of girlie magazines, has shown little inventiveness in its ingredients, confining itself to "Spanish fly" and inferior ginseng at superior prices. One company offers a line of "Potent Placebo Aphrodisiacs" with names as boring as their effects: Virility Pills, Prolong Pills, Stay Hard Pills, Erection Pills, and Hard-on Pills. Others have expended much ingenuity at least on the name, making the ads into a sort of concrete poesy.

> *Buy Renox, Stimulol, Vice Spice, Passion-Plus,*
> *   Peter Power, Turn-On, and Vita-Pep at "Pills Are Us":*
> *We have Mono, Heureka, Sexine, The Real McCoy,*
> *   Amor Star, Love in a Jar, or Creme de Joy.*
> *Get your Okasa Lozenges, your Anal-Eze,*
> *   Your Fakir's Pills and Pills of Hercules.*
> *Who'll be the first for Testacoids and Pearls of Titus,*
> *   Dynamin, Samson, Dragees de Venus?*
> *Don't forget some Remogland and Para-Mate.*
> *   Send your money now before it's too late.*

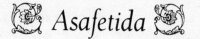# Asafetida

THE dried juice of a plant of the Iranian-Afghani plateau, asafetida ("stinking gum") is the coprophiliac's aphrodisiac. Its odor is often politely described as garlicky, but it is much closer to feces. Asafetida was called Devil's Dung in the belief that Satan scattered his body over the earth as herbage to illustrate the darker side of the Doctrine of Signatures. When the herb is fresh the smell is so commanding, the taste so bitter—and behind it all lurks such an elusive rotten sweetness, reminiscent of innermost secrets—that one can almost understand a taste for it. It is sometimes burned for incense. It is used in Worcestershire sauce. When dried and much diluted with flour, the resin still stinks but goes surprisingly well with beans, as Indians and Pakistanis know, who call it *hing* and *laser*.

The yellowish red gum is a stimulant tonic to the alimentary mucous membrane, once much used for dyspepsia, flatulence, colic, and constipation. Since it is quite safe it was preferred for children, although who knows what hatreds its taste may have begun. Since the volatile oil is eliminated through the lungs, asafetida also found favor among herbalists as an expectorant for use in asthma, bronchitis, and coughs.

In the parts of Asia where it is used, asafetida has some fame as an aphrodisiac. This may be due to some effect on the brain exerted by its ferulic acid or umbelliferone, but herbals are evenly divided as to whether it is a stimulant or a sedative. It increases pulse and blood pressure slightly, and creates a sensation of bodily warmth without an actual rise in temperature.

Asafetida can be made into an emulsion by boiling an ounce in a pint of water. A tablespoon of this is the average dose. It is also available as a tincture, taken ½–1 teaspoon at a time. Perhaps the best method is to take it as a powder pressed into pills of 3–20 grains (.2–1.3 grams) to bypass the taste. In the United States it is most commonly seen at herb shops and Indian groceries in the form of a powder or hard globs of resin, both much diluted with flour and gum arabic.

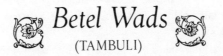

# Betel Wads
## (TAMBULI)

PICTURE the ideal summer job. Freed from school and wearing the tropical minimum, boys and girls wander among the majestic palms. They spend long hours in raucous games, quiet talk, and fervid explorations of the still-unfamiliar reaches of each other's anatomies. After biorefreshment and a bit of rest, they climb the betel palms, inhale the fragrant ivory blossoms, and, their baskets full of the egglike orange fruit, return to earth anon for another round of dip-the-wick.

Such is the hard life of those who gather the *pinang* of Malaya, the *supari* of India, known to us as the areca or betel nut, one of the world's most popular stimulants. The brown conical seeds that lie within the orange fruit are dried and combined with several other ingredients to form what in 1930 was estimated by Louis Lewin to be the drug of choice for 200 million Asians. It serves them as an energizer, euphoriant, and aphrodisiac, the ideal accompaniment to the idyllic harvest.

This pickup is a wad or cud of five ingredients, sucked or chewed for hours. Foremost are thin slices of the areca nut itself, which grows in many parts of tropical Asia. The seed releases four alkaloids (arecoline, arecain, guracine, and arecaidine). The primary one is arecoline, a central nervous system stimulant that also temporarily increases the pumping efficiency of the heart.

To the wad are added a pinch of burnt lime (hydrated calcium oxide) for the proper pH to release arecoline into the saliva and a sprinkle of catechu gum or gambier, obtained from the *Acacia catechu* vine, rich in astringent tannic acid that keeps the flow of saliva from becoming excessive. The mixture is flavored with a bit of cardamom, nutmeg, or clove and wrapped in a leaf from the betel pepper (*Piper chavica* or *P. betel*), which gives its name (*tambuli* or *pahn* in India) to the entire morsel. Betel leaf is itself a mild stimulant, saliva promoter, and breath sweetener for amorous messages.

Don't mistake me. The effects of this little tidbit are perhaps milder than the popular myth suggests and are a general stimulant rather than a direct aphrodisiac. Still, it is one of those blessings that increases the level of happiness in the world if used in moderation. Overindulgence can make one dizzy, nauseous, diarrheal, and even convulsive. Long-term overuse (not uncommon) stains the mouth permanently red and probably leads to an eventual decrease in sexual interest. But this noble concoction is well worth an occasional crimson grin; it can sometimes be found in the United States in Indian grocery stores.

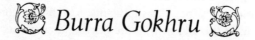 *Burra Gokhru*

THE seeds, fruit, and fresh leaves of *Pedalium murex* (whose native name is variously anglicized as *bada gokeroo* or *burra gokhru*) is used in India as a soothing diuretic for genitourinary infections. For impotence and excessive nocturnal emissions, a pint of weak infusion of the seeds is used. A stronger solution can be made by crushing one part seeds to twenty parts water (by weight, 1 ounce to 1.2 pints), steeping them for a day, then straining the liquid and adding an ounce or two of grain alcohol (or 2 jiggers vodka) as a preservative. This can be taken in doses of one teaspoon three times a day. This plant has been little studied in the West, but it may stimulate the genital ganglia, much as damiana or yohimbé, only milder.

# 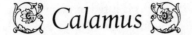 Calamus

CALAMUS is one of the best-known herbs in the world, growing in marshes throughout the Northern Hemisphere and familiar to all peoples as an aromatic appetizer and dispeller of gas. The fragrant roots are bactericidal and good for alimentary canal infections. They impressed Walt Whitman as a "token of comrades" and under such names as sweet flag, sweet sedge, and galingale they show up in perfumes, snuff, gin, bitters, candies, and as a sweet carpet on the floors of cathedrals. Several American Indian tribes used the roots for toothaches, colds, and abortions; East Indian mothers so often used *bacha* tea for baby's colic that severe fines were levied on druggists who refused to open up shop in the middle of the night and sell it.

In Arabia, Iran, and India, calamus also has a reputation as a daily aid for lengthening life, tightening memory, and raising libido. One Indian recipe combines two ounces of the dried root with a dram of coriander and half a dram of black pepper in a pint of water boiled down to twelve ounces. Back on the other side of the world, the Cree Indians of Alberta chewed a two-inch, pencil-thick stick daily as a sexual nerve tonic. Indirect evidence indicated that longer pieces were used as psychedelics. The root's volatile oil contains enough hallucinogenic $\alpha$- and $\beta$-asarone to make ten-inch segments a potent way to alter consciousness. How these substances work and what gonadic effects calamus has are still not known.

# 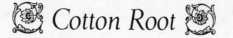 Cotton Root

A DECOCTION of the inner root bark of the short-stapled cotton (*Gossypium herbaceum*) is listed in many herbals as a remedy for "sexual lassitude" in both sexes. I have not found any analysis of how it works other than Mrs. Grieve's enigmatic note in *A Modern Herbal* that it contains "a peculiar acid resin" which quickly deteriorates and turns red on exposure to oxygen. I've tried it without noticing any effect, but am holding some in reserve in case an attack of lassitude develops.

Cotton root is more commonly women's medicine. It's used to bring on a delayed menstruation, to treat uterine hemorrhage caused by fibroid tumors, and as a weaker but less dangerous substitute for ergot* in promoting labor and inducing abortion. For these purposes cotton root was used by slaves in the antebellum South. The usual recipe is four ounces of the root bark boiled in a quart of water until the liquid is reduced to a pint, and one wineglass (4 ounces) of it taken every half hour. If its action is indeed similar to ergot, this amount and frequency may be excessive.

---

* Ergot (*Claviceps purpurea*, or rye smut) is a fungus that digests and replaces grains of rye, forming enlarged crooked spurs in the ears of the grain. It contains ergotamine tartrate, a powerful vasoconstrictor which is sometimes used to relieve migraines and from which LSD is synthesized. Another alkaloid, ergonovine, makes ergot a strong oxytocic (an agent that induces uterine contractions). European midwives and doctors sometimes used it to bring on labor or abortion, but it is dangerous. Other compounds in it, such as ergotoxin, can cause gangrene; and ergot poisoning, once common in Europe's rye bread country, results in a sometimes fatal, hyperactive delirium called St. Anthony's Fire.

# 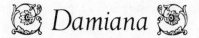 Damiana

THE ancient Aztecs used this herb as a tonic, aphrodisiac, and cure for impotence, but most of their knowledge of the plant disappeared during the zealous persecution by Spanish missionaries. Fortunately, damiana was not altogether forgotten; modern lovers are rediscovering its potential and creating their own traditions.

Also called shepherd's herb and stag's herb, known to Indians as *xmisibcoc* and to botanists as *Turnera diffusa* or *Turnera aphrodisiaca*, damiana is a small shrub native to the American Southwest, Mexico, and the West Indies. A compound called damianin produces both a bitter taste and direct stimulation of the nerves and sexual organs. A volatile, greenish oil that smells like chamomile may aid in the herb's activity.

Damianin is chemically related to strychnine (see page 191), with the advantage strychnine lacks—safety. An active dose of strychnine allows nerve messages to spread out undirectedly throughout the nervous system. The stimulus is unbearable, causing uncontrollable convulsions or death from overstimulation of the heart. Damianin has a similar but much milder effect on nerve sensitivity, with a large margin of safety. Still, in Mexico, nux vomica, the plant source of strychnine, is sometimes mixed with damiana to heighten its effect.

In the 1930s several livestock breeders were using damiana to stimulate their studs, a fact which led sexologist George Ryley Scott to try it. He pronounced it, after "extensive experiments, quite useless," but did not mention how he prepared it. He may have used too little or may not have taken it continuously over a long enough period. Philadelphia doctor W. H. Myers, after extensive use of it in cases of sexual debility, pronounced it ". . . the most effective and only remedy that in my hands had a successful result in all cases," using fifteen to thirty drops of fluid extract per day.

The last decade's resurgence of interest in herbs has brought damiana back, if not to popularity, at least to the realm of available knowledge. A tea is usually prepared with one or two tablespoons of the dried leaves steeped in a pint of hot water. Some people also smoke the leaves, but the herb is so harsh on the throat that a water pipe is usually needed. The smoke in combination with the tea gives a faint marijuanalike high, *too* faint to be worthwhile.

Word of mouth has it that damiana has a stronger effect on women, but both sexes tell of erotic dreams when they drink a cup before bedtime and increased sensitivity when they take it before balling. The effect is cumulative, growing more noticeable after a few days. Personally I noted no change in my dream content and no immediate effects after each cup. But a marked rise in the lust level was unmistakable after four or five days, especially from the cordial recipe given below. Upping the dose beyond a cup or two per day does not seem to increase the effect, however, and prolonged overuse (many cups daily) is suspected of causing liver damage. But a cup a day is a definite sensual turn-on with no known side effects.

Once available only through such herbal pharmacies as Kiehl's in New York City, damiana is now marketed by many herb companies by mail order or through health-food stores. It is often blended with saw palmetto berries (see page 140) for an even stronger boost.

Louis T. Culling, in his *Manual of Sex Magic*, describes his sexual rejuvenation after two weeks of damiana tea every evening. To make his tea, Culling simmered two heaping tablespoons of the dried herb in one large cup of water for five minutes; he drank an extra cup before—ideally, starting a few days before—coitus. Culling called damiana a "communicative" aphrodisiac as well as a physical one. He and friends who tested it found that ". . . people who would ordinarily have conversed with us quite casually were unusually friendly, even to the point of intimate interest." He kept a diary of his test of damiana during an affair at age sixty-nine with a young Tijuana waitress. At one point he writes:

> Last night was like being in an Arabian Nights' story. Four times was La Encantadora taken on the magic carpet to the mountain of ecstasy. Three times I sailed with her—already an incredible exploit for me. Yet she has said that she is going to be with me again the coming afternoon and night! It is time for that feeling of complete surfeit. Yet I am looking forward to this with an enchanted imagination that rivals the anticipation of the first love affair of my youth.

Culling also mentions a damiana cordial imported from Mexico, called Liqueur for Lovers. This, however, contains too little of the herb to be effective.

The following recipe has been circulating in the California underground for a few years, and first surfaced in Adam Gottlieb's excellent *Sex Drugs and Aphrodisiacs*.

> Soak 1 ounce of dried damiana in a pint of vodka for 5 days. Pass the liquid through a coffee filter, then steep the vodka-sodden leaves in spring or distilled water (chlorinated tap water will affect the taste) for another 5 days. Filter as before. Then warm the water extract and mix with ½–1 cup honey. Keep the temperature under 160° F. or the honey's flavor will also begin to deteriorate. Combine the two solutions. Drink it as is or age it for a few weeks. A cordial glass of it makes a delicious and sexy nightcap.

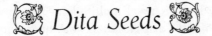

# Dita Seeds

THE bark of this seventy-foot east Asian tree has been used for ages from India to the Philippines as a remedy for painful menstrual cramps, fevers, and dyspepsia. These properties are thought to be due to ditamine ($C_{16}H_{19}NO_2$), and other alkaloids, but only the seeds contain another substance, chlorogenine ($C_{21}H_{20}N_2O_4$), reportedly a powerful aphrodisiac, at least in men. Its action has not been much studied, but it allegedly helps maintain a hard erection and prevent premature ejaculation. As different batches of seeds may vary in potency, it is wise to start with a small dose, about two grams, and increase the amount if needed. The crushed seeds are soaked in water overnight, and the strained liquid is drunk the next day.

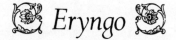

# Eryngo

IF THE root of the sea holly (*Eryngium maritimum*) still holds any of its former fame as a love food, the echo comes from the ample mouth of Falstaff, who implores, "Let the sky rain potatoes, let it thunder to the tune of Greensleeves, hail kissing comfits and stone eringoes: let there be a tempest of provocation. . . ." The comfits were candied holly roots, widely used in England before and after Shakespeare to renew the aged, conserve the wasted, and fortify the young. The confections made by the seventeenth-century apothecary Robert Burton in his factory at Colchester were the most sought after and were credited with the most marvelous cures after a sample he sent to Court was ecstatically received.

The Greeks had eaten the young asparaguslike shoots and the roots. The plant's name comes from the Greek verb for "to eruct" (belch or fart), for the root provides some relief for gas problems. This was probably its main use among the Romans, although the gullible Pliny lists his usual multitude of ailments it can cure. "Applied with salted axle-grease and wax ointment it heals scrofulous sores, parotid tumors, superficial abscesses, and the falling away of the flesh from the bones; fractures, too." Called "hundred heads" for its thistlelike flower balls, it is also one of the numberless plants Pliny touts for snakebite, as well as (without batting an eye) frogbite. He also mentions the legend of Phaon, the boatman of Lesbos who won Sappho's love by finding an eryngo root shaped like a penis.

Modern herbalists who have not forgotten it entirely sometimes use a decoction of eryngo as a diuretic or expectorant for kidney, bladder, or lung infections. A decoction of it is very bitter and astringent, with a strong drying effect on the mucous membranes.

The chemistry of the sea holly is unexplored. The bitter and slightly aromatic essences can be dissolved by boiling two teaspoons of the small rootlets or the broken main roots for five minutes in a cup of water. The ingredients can also be extracted, perhaps more efficiently, by soaking the roots in wine as the ancients did, or in something of a modern proof. For those who prefer to try the Elizabethan sweets, which taste a bit like candied angelica, here is a recipe from John Gerard's 1597 *Herbal.*

*Use only the thick sections of the main root, not the tiny rootlets. Boil the roots for 4 hours or until soft. Peel them and draw the central pith out the end; if necessary, split the roots and cut out the pith. Combine 1 pound sugar, 1 egg white, and 1 pint water; boil and skim the scum. After this mixture has become a thick syrup, take it off the heat; as it cools add a few tablespoons rosewater, 1 tablespoon water [or ½ teaspoon dried cinnamon] and 1 grain of musk [or a dab of genuine musk oil]. Soak the roots in this syrup for 1 day. Then heat the mixture again for an hour, stirring occasionally, but do not let it boil. Remove the roots, place them on sugar-dusted paper, and leave them in a warm place to harden.*

This procedure is fine for the thick roots, up to several feet long, which Gerard gathered and that can still be found in sandy English seashore soil or in private rock gardens. But when using the puny finger-sized knobs of commercial eryngo, there is no sense being too finicky about manicuring or one is left with nothing but a pile of peel and pith. Perhaps small roots lack something that only develops as they grow larger. Mine had a coating of sweet, fragrant nostalgia, resolving to a horrible bitterness inside. I'm afraid the candies' appeal lies in the flavorings, not in the root. They serve only to remind us of a time when sugar was considered good for you.

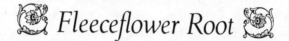 *Fleeceflower Root*

THE smoke-dried tubers of *Polygonum multiflorum* are one of the favorite tonics of Chinese herbal medicine. Oriental doctors say their *ho shou niao* nourishes most of the essential organ systems, including nerves, muscles, bones, viscera, and glands, but its primary use is to build up the blood's oxygen capacity. It is about half starch and 3.7 percent lecithin, with traces of an alcohol called chrysophanol.

Fleeceflower tuber can occasionally be found in this country in powder form, which makes preparation a simple matter of boiling a teaspoon or more (7–15 grams) in a cup of water for a few minutes. Otherwise the rocklike spud must be wrapped in a cloth and cracked with a hammer or boiled for an hour or two until it can be mashed, boiled some more (or puréed in a blender), and strained. Powder or broken pieces can be steeped in spirits for a week or so, then filtered for an alcohol extract. Like all tonics, fleeceflower's effects are gradual and take at least a week or two to become noticeable. The bitter root is a safe, gentle fortifier but should not be combined with garlic or iron supplements.

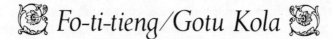

# Fo-ti-tieng/Gotu Kola

THE most famous advocate of fo-ti-tieng died in 1933, and disbelief of the claims made for his life may be one reason why this herb is still so little known in the United States. Chinese herbalist Li Ch'ung-yun was, according to Chinese government records, born in 1677, making him an exceedingly well-preserved 256 when he died.

Whether we choose to believe this statistic or not, Li certainly lived a long time; he kept his own hair and teeth sound and his twenty-fourth wife happy to the end. He said, "Sit like a tortoise, walk like a pigeon, and sleep like a dog. Fast regularly and, except for ginseng, eat nothing but vegetables that grow in the sunlight." Beyond this advice, he imputed part of his amazing vitality to his daily ration of *Hydrocotyle asiatica minor*, sometimes called elephant's-foot, a low, spreading marsh plant of southern Asia.

Botanists do not agree whether gotu kola, sometimes named *Centella asiatica*, is merely a geographical variant of fo-ti-tieng. Its effects and folklore are similar. It grows wild in marshes of India, Sri Lanka, and southern Africa.

A Sinhalese gotu proverb claims, "Two leaves a day keep old age away." An Indian anecdote reported in the West tells of an aging female elephant at Deshapur who gained a new lease on life and bore a calf after gotu kola leaves were added to her diet. The fresh leaves of both plants are held superior to the dried herb, but except in Hawaii and along the Gulf Coast, the plants must be grown indoors in this country. They need shade, warmth, and abundant moisture. Dried leaves and extracts are available by mail from many herb companies and from some health-food stores (usually in capsule form). Prices now average five dollars to eight dollars per pound. Fo-ti-tieng is more expensive, over three dollars an ounce.

A daily cup of tea made with one to two teaspoons of either herb is an excellent tonic for the brain, nerves, and hormone systems. It conduces to proper digestion, and possibly to resistance of disease and aging. Amounts of one to two tablespoons daily give a gradual but pronounced boost to sexual vitality, especially when energy has been on the wane.

The amount of scientific research done on these intriguing plants can only be described as pitiful. French biochemist Jules Lepine has isolated a yet unnamed substance which showed a regenerative effect on nerve and endocrine tissue. His work was confirmed by Professor Menier of the Académie Scientifique, who called it vitamin X. Other tests have hinted that this compound affects part of the adrenal glands, which helps rid the body of toxins. These tentative results tally with the claim of Indian pandit Nanddo Narian, who at age 107 told his chelas that gotu kola provides a missing nutrient without which humans can never be free of disease.

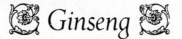

# Ginseng

WE OWE our enjoyment of Asiatic ginseng today to the nineteenth-century Chinese emperor Tao Kuang, who put strict controls on its use when it was in danger of extinction. American and Asian types of *Panax* have been used since unremembered time as a fortifying medicine. The Meskwaki Indian women of Wisconsin mixed ginseng, mica, gelatin, and snake meat to make a "bagging agent" for getting husbands. One of the many Chinese ginseng tonics calls for:

> *3 liang (108 grams) of ginseng, ginger, and p'ai chu (Atractylis ovata). Cook them in 8 sheng (about 8 quarts) of water, boil it down to 5 quarts, and drink 1 quart a day in three doses.*

Commercial-quality ginseng costs between five and fifteen dollars an ounce, so this mixture must at least stimulate the energy to make the money involved.

Ginseng and a close relative with similar effects, Siberian ginseng (*Eleutherococcus senticosus*) have been intensely studied in the past few years, first in the Soviet Union and now in the United States. Both plants have several sterone compounds that work as mild anabolic (body-building) stimulants. Anabolics increase the body's energy output, as opposed to catabolic (body-wasting) stimulants like cocaine, which mobilize energy already stored. Ginseng has shown itself to be so good at preventing damage from stress of all kinds that a new word was coined for it: adaptogen. *Eleutherococcus* is slightly stronger, as well as more abundant, but *Panax* also contains panoxic acid, a mixture of unsaturated fatty acids that aids proper use of cholesterol; ginsenin, an insulinlike material; panaxin, a central nervous system stimulant; and panaquilon, which may be an endocrine tonic.

A daily gram or so of the dried root, or a slug of an extract like the traditional Shaosing wine, is one of the best efficiency herbs known. Except in large doses, no effects are apparent until one suddenly looks back on a surprisingly productive day. Ginseng can be a fine indirect tonic aphrodisiac but is not known to have any direct influence on sexual response.

Then, too, ginseng may not be as good for the average American as it is for the average Asian. Unlike Western medicine, the Chinese healing art subordinates its facts and theories to a unifying philosophical concept—the interplay of *yang* and *yin*. This is a universal pattern of push-pull, tension-release, positive-negative, energy-matter duality, seen as operating on all levels, from galactic clusters to subatomic particles. Health is conceived as a dynamic balance between similar forces in the body.

Yang represents the "solar" or "male" factors of light, warmth, fullness, dryness, and stimulation, which, with the sympathetic nervous system and acid-reacting food, are manifested by slower digestion, faster pulse, dilation of the pupil of the eye, constriction of blood vessels, cold extremities, and increased wakefulness. Yin represents the "lunar" or "female" factors of darkness, coldness, emptiness, moisture, and preservation, which, with the parasympathetic nervous system and alkaline-reacting food, are manifested by faster digestion, slower pulse, contraction of the pupil of the eye, dilation of blood vessels, warm extremities, languor, drowsiness, meditation, sleep, and dreams.

Doctors familiar with *jen-shen* ("man-root") remind us that it is a very strong yang medicine. It is a poor choice for the many Westerners already unbalanced in this direction, especially for heavy users of coffee or other stimulants.

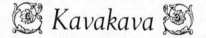 *Kavakava*

KAVAKAVA or *ava ava* or *yangona* is an intoxicating drink made from the roots of a shrub pepper (*Piper methysticum*) that grows on most of the South Pacific islands from Hawaii south to Polynesia and west to New Guinea. Today it is primarily brewed in water as a mildly stimulating tea, but when treated so as to release its full complement of resins and alkaloids, soluble only in oil or alcohol, it is a potent narcotic. By affecting mainly the spinal nerves, it produces an exquisitely warm somatic drowsiness which usually ends in sleep but leaves the mind alert for one-half to two hours.

Once a major part of the islanders' ceremonies, the kava was emulsified by chewing the lilac-scented but bitterly soapy-tasting root for hours, then mixing it with coconut milk. For Westerners who consider this way unnecessarily hard on the taste buds, here's a variant method:

> Take 1 ounce chopped or ground kava and mix in a
> blender with 2 tablespoons coconut or other oil, 1 table-

*spoon lecithin, and a cup or more water or coconut milk. Serves 2–4.*

The active resins can also be extracted in grain or isopropyl alcohol, then dried by evaporation in a water bath or double boiler. A small pill of this resin can then be taken dissolved in warm brandy or vodka.

Kava is not much of an aphrodisiac because of its depression of bodily nerve function. Those interested in further study should consult E. F. Steinmetz's monograph. Kava was long tested as a local anesthetic, however, and one experiment with this property is worth trying in the bedroom. When placed on the glans of penis or clitoris, the extracted resin or an oil emulsion effects a tingling numbness of the surface nerve-endings. Milder and somehow warmer than cocaine or opium put to the same end, kava applied by hand or tongue can afford the man more relaxed control of ejaculation and both sexes a slow buildup of charge in the deeper fibers before orgasm.

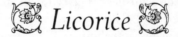 *Licorice*

*Glycyrrhiza* ("sweet root") species are known all over the world as one of the best medicines to soothe a cough or sore throat; their juices helped make the Smith Brothers rich and children blacktongued and happy. Some older cultures also found that the roots make a fine ingredient for restorative and mild aphrodisiacs. The Chinese trusted their *kan ts'ao* as a lung and stomach tonic. The Scythian nomads, who introduced the Greeks to the delicious roots growing by Lake Maeotis (Sea of Azov), could live for fortnight marches on nothing but mare's-milk cheese and strong licorice tea.

In India, a favorite *kama*-time drink was made with licorice,

milk, and honey much like the one Nicholas Culpeper describes
in his herbals of the mid seventeenth century:

> Place ½–1 pound chopped dried root in 3 pints water;
> boil down to 1 quart, then strain. The decoction can be
> taken cold or hot with milk and honey to taste.

A weaker, less mucilaginous tea requires one to two teaspoons per
cup. If available, the juice of the fresh roots is even sweeter.

Licorice figures prominently in one of the oldest herbal recipes known, a popular beverage of ancient Egypt, *mai sus*. In fact,
King Tutankhamun was sent on his eternal voyage with a store of
(among other things) licorice root. The drink, in one version, goes
like this:

> Crush 1 ounce each licorice root, sesame seeds, and
> fennel seeds in a mortar. Boil them in 1 pint water rap-
> idly for 5 minutes, then reduce heat, cover, and simmer
> for 20 minutes more. Let stand until cool, then strain.

Licorice's main ingredient is glycyrrhizin, a sweet mixture of
salts of glycyrrhizic acid. There is also some sugar, starch, a little
protein, and asparagine. Analysis in 1950 showed that licorice
contains estrogenic substances, but how well they are assimilated
and how they affect the human libido have not been determined.

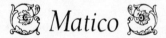 *Matico*

THIS eight-foot-tall pepper (*Piper angustifolium*) is native to Peru
and Ecuador, but now grows in many rainy parts of Latin
America. It gets its name from the Spanish soldier, Mateo, who

became the first European to use its blood-clotting quality when wounded in Peru; hence its nickname, soldier's herb. The Indians call it *thoho-thoho* or *moho-moho*, and they use it as an aphrodisiac and general stimulant. A tablespoon of the dried leaves are boiled for a minute in a cup of water, then left to steep for half an hour. The drink is then strained and served cold.

It feels like just another mildly stimulating diuretic to me, and Western herbalists have adopted the herb as such, usually in a weaker tea or 50- to 75-grain doses of the powder.

Matico contains an aromatic volatile oil (giving it its sagelike odor and styptic properties), potassium nitrate (saltpeter), and other salts, and a compound called maticine, which may be the same as the artanthic acid named in earlier sources. Perhaps it is this on which any stimulation from matico depends.

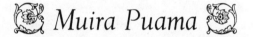

# Muira Puama

THE inner bark and wood of the South American tree *Lyriosma ovata* are known to the natives of the upper Amazon and Orinoco as *muira puama*. The Jivaro and other tribes chew the fresh plant or boil it fresh or dried to make a nerve stimulant and tonic aphrodisiac.

In the last two or three decades, muira puama has passed from the jungle to the rest of Brazilian society and is often sold by American herb dealers. It has been admitted to the Brazilian pharmacopoeia as a remedy for impotence. It is used externally as a strong decoction rubbed on the genitals and is considered a central nervous system tonic and appetite enhancer. The fluid extract is given in daily doses of fifteen to twenty drops; no side effects have been observed in practice so far.

In the early 1960s the German firm of E. Scheurich had included muira puama in its "Josual," a rejuvenation product used by Latin American doctors; other ingredients were testicular tissue, anterior pituitary extract, lecithin, cola extract, yohimbine hydrochloride, calcium lactate, and strychnine. Muira puama is now a common over- or under-the-counter sex aid throughout Latin America, and it is becoming better known in the United States.

Good chemical analyses and controlled medical experiments on the plant are still lacking, but the active substances reside in a resin that is imperfectly extracted in water but fully soluble in alcohol. Hence recipes for use differ widely from source to source. The powdered root can simply be packed in size 00 gelatin capsules, of which six are taken per day. Two to four tablespoons, or up to an ounce, of the shaved or powdered wood can be boiled in water for fifteen minutes. A cup of this decoction is supposed to have gratifying effects when drunk an hour or two before lovemaking, but don't make it too strong the first time. Instead of a gentle heat, too much at once lights a disconcerting blaze in the gut and on the skin, and one tends more toward aggravated restlessness.

Alcohol extraction delivers more of the crucial ingredients but also modifies the effect with the booze, which may be a problem for those especially sensitive to it. The same amount, four tablespoons (about an ounce), of the herb can be steeped in two cups of vodka, brandy, or overproof rum for two weeks. Shake the brew daily, then strain it and drink a shot or two per day. A faster method is to place the herb in liquor that is gently boiling in a double boiler or on a hot plate with variable control. Care must be taken to keep the alcohol from igniting. The process can be repeated with the same batch of herb to take out all the resin. If pure grain (ethyl) or isopropyl alcohol is used, it can be evaporated to obtain the pure resin, of which a pea-sized pellet or less can be dissolved on the tongue.

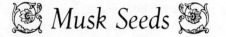 # Musk Seeds

Too many allegedly erotic herbs have a sexless taste, but musk seeds are a happy exception. They come from an evergreen shrub (*Abelmoschus* or *Hibiscus moschatus*) native to tropical Asia and the East Indies and now cultivated in India, Egypt, and the West Indies as well. Also known as amber seed, abelmosk, and ambrette, the seeds grow in a capsule shaped like a five-cornered pyramid and look like delicately striped gray-brown snail shells the size of a lentil or smaller. True to their name, they smell and taste of musk and are sometimes chewed to sweeten the mouth. Much of the crop goes to the perfume industry, but the Arabs use some to flavor coffee. The seeds make a delicious brew and combine just as well with chocolate.

Folk medicine considers musk seeds to be a mild nerve calmative and aphrodisiac, probably because of the intoxicating aroma. The seeds are usually ground and brewed into an emulsion with water or milk. In India a concentrated tincture is most often used for flavoring.


# Night-blooming Cereus

This fleshy cactus (*Cereus* or *Selenicereus grandiflorus*) of the southwestern United States, Mexico, and Jamaica does indeed have grand flowers. Up to a foot across, they smell sweetly of vanilla on the night they open, but dry up and die after only six hours. The root has a long tradition of use among the Indians. Known commercially as cactus flowers, the blooms and, more especially, the flower stems are the parts used today by herbalists and homeopaths. They serve for various heart ailments, including palpitations, angina pectoris, and cardiac neuralgia, as well as menstrual headaches and inflammation of the prostate or bladder.

They are not coital excitants, but the flowers have been useful in some cases of sexual inability due to exhaustion. To this end the best form to use is two to ten drops of the fresh juice. Alternatively, one-half gram of the fresh stems may be chewed, or combined with liquor since the active ingredient is readily soluble in alcohol. Most of the problems for which this herb is used are serious, so consult a trustworthy doctor before using it. As always, when first taking a potent herb, start at the low end of the dosage range. Results of an excess of Cereus range from stomach irritation to delirium.

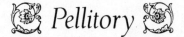 *Pellitory*

SPANISH pellitory (*Anacyclus pyrethrum*, formerly called *Anthemis pyrethrum*) is a small perennial of the Mediterranean region that looks somewhat like chamomile. It is not to be confused with two other herbs sometimes given the same name: several types of Chrysanthemum collectively called feverfew, pyrethron, or Persian pellitory, and whose dried flower buds are powdered and used as an insecticide because they are harmless to humans; and various Parietaria species named pellitory-of-the-wall, one of the best herbs for kidney stones.

Spanish pellitory, also known as herb Bertram, was used as a love stimulant chiefly by the ancient Romans. As a means of quickly raising the flag again, Ovid speaks of pellitory root steeped in wine just long enough to caution against it. He lists it with Spanish fly as a dangerous irritant. This is hard to confirm directly; the herb has gone out of use, except in India, and does not grow in the United States.

Ovid's warning is probably to the point. Henry Lyte's 1578 translation of *Dodoens' Niewe Herball or Historie of Plantes* calls the root "hoate and dry in the thirde degree." It continued in use a few centuries more as a local counterirritant for pains of neuralgia and toothache. Culpeper's praise for it as "one of the best purges of the brain" is hardly reassuring, and the only analysis I've found showed many nutrient minerals and a salivary stimulant, pyrethrin, but also a brown acrid oil. At one time the Arabs made it into an ointment with ginger and lilac, rubbing it in for extra heat, but it doesn't sound ingestible.

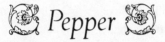 *Pepper*

*Brother, I had to fill this belly, and when I did,*
*I put a whole cellar full of pepper on my steak,*
*for Aphrodite, what the hell you call it.*
*And now I'm rarin'. I'm like asbestos all inside. . . .*
*Yeah and I'm all rarin'.*
—JAMES T. FARRELL, from *Gas House McGinty*

IN THE Lisimbu initiation rites for girls of the Kuta tribes of northern Okondia in pre-Colonial Africa, a mother had to hold her daughter's head close over a fire on which a handful of pepper had been thrown. The young woman-to-be then had to improvise her own personal erotic dance and crawl between her mother's legs in token of rebirth as a sexual adult.

All the many *Piper* and *Capsicum* plants commonly called pepper are distinguished by burning volatile oils. Except in enormous amounts they do no actual damage, but merely stimulate the heat-sensing nerves of skin and mucous membrane. The sensation of these irritants in the gut and urethra gives false but sometimes still effective aphrodisiac heat. Much use is made of this sensation in Asia, where Chinese men drink cubeb tea and Arabs mix it with honey. (A black pepper alkaloid called piperine, consisting of the same atoms $[C_{17}H_{19}NO_3]$ as morphine in a slightly different arrangement, may modulate the warmth of the oils in a way as yet unknown.) However, unless the vanadium in black pepper turns out to be a stimulating mineral, we must look elsewhere for true heat.

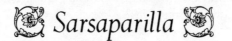 *Sarsaparilla*

SARSAPARILLA still smells of spiffy white summer suits, wrought-iron ice-cream-parlor chairs, and handlebar moustaches. Back when root beer was made with roots, sarsaparilla was one of them. It was commonly sold as a spring tonic, blood purifier, and restorer of lost manhood. A Spanish doctor named Monardes introduced it to white man's medicine in 1568 after studying the Indians' use of it as a fortifier and remedy for syphilis, for which it was used until the advent of arsenicals.

Native Americans from Mexico to the Andes had valued various species of *Smilax* in treating impotence and sexual debility of old age. The beginning of World War II overshadowed the 1939 discovery of raw materials for sex hormones in sarsaparilla. Dr. Emerick Solmo, a Budapest chemist living in Mexico, found that the well-known root bark contains sterones. Today sarsaparilla is the chief commercial source of testosterone, the "male" secretion that grows beards and fully developed penises, but is also essential to muscle tone and sexual drive in *both* sexes. The plant also yields sarsasapogenin for making the female hormone progesterone. Synthetic cortin, an adrenal hormone that defends us against infection and depression, also starts from sarsaparilla.

Older herbals recommend a simple tea in which the root bark's effects are too weak to be felt. A modern recipe, first promulgated by Adam Gottlieb, is a sure but perhaps temporary cure for lax libido caused by hormonal insufficiency.

> Simmer 2–3 heaping tablespoons (up to ½ ounce) of the shaved inner root bark for 5 or 10 minutes in 1 pint of water. Be careful it doesn't boil over, as the saponins will create a head of foam. Drink 1–2 cups (up to 1 pint) of this decoction morning and evening, swirling each sip around the mouth, as the sterones are best ad-sorbed through the mucous membrane.
>
> An excellent homemade tincture can also be pre-pared by using a bottle half full of sarsaparilla and filling it up with equal parts water and grain alcohol—or vodka. Let it stand two weeks, shaking it well each day. Take a tablespoon four to five times a day.

Oddly enough, sarsaparilla will not make an already lusty person much lustier; it may eventually decrease desire. External sources of hormones tend to signal the body to shut down its own internal factories. Therefore this remedy should not be continued beyond a couple of weeks. The idea is to support lazy glands, spark them into renewed life, rather than become dependent on a substitute.

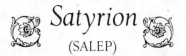

# Satyrion
## (SALEP)

ORCHIS, a son of passion (he was the offspring of a nymph and a satyr), was drunk. Singing and dancing among the other cele-brants of the vintage festival to honor Bacchus, he couldn't tell the difference between one of the god's virgin priestesses and the other young bacchantes, but he was not too far gone to be bowled over by her beauty. Apparently she was also wined enough to forget her station, for she went along with his seduction—or maybe it was an abduction. Any cries she might have made would have been drowned in the shouting, and soon she was neither maid nor priestess.

The pious locals were so outraged that they tore Orchis to pieces and scattered his body about the meadows. His father begged the gods to put him back together again, but in council they agreed that if he were so intemperate the world was better off without him. But they were moved enough by a father's grief to decree that all of his parts should return each spring as the flowers that bear his name—orchids.

True to his ballsy nature, the herb Orchis became had two bulbous roots, each shaped like an *orchis* (Greek for testicle), and because the orchids were such strong aphrodisiacs they must be owned by servants of the lust-god Pan, hence grown from a satyr's son or, in an alternate myth, a satyr's semen.

Satyrion's feats were literally incredible. In Book Nine of his *Enquiry into Plants*, Theophrastus tells of a specimen sent as a gift to Antiochus, King of Syria. So potent was its very aura that the delivery slave was able to screw seventy times in a row just from holding the plant in his hand, only stopping when his cock began to bleed. God knows what Antiochus did after ingesting the stuff. In a similar vein, a certain Proculus allegedly made love with a hundred women in fifteen days, and Hercules repaid the gracious hospitality of Thespius by laboring on fifty of his once-virgin daughters after a drink of orchis.

Since no one seems to get such results anymore, there has been much dispute about the exact identity of this herb. These legends, especially the one about Antiochus's slave, sound like the excruciating satyriasis of Spanish fly, but various orchids' fame persists (with gradually diminishing scorecards) down to the present.

Many orchids were used, but they fall into two types, based

on the shape of their tubers. Some have a pair of elongated, branched roots; the more highly prized types have a round, testicle-shaped pair. In most cases one root is larger and plumper than the other. Dioscorides says the larger tuber of red orchid or butterfly orchid helps men beget males; the smaller one, he says, aids women in conceiving females. Thessalian wise women, the ancient world's most sought-after witches, prescribed the softer, large one in goat's milk as an aphrodisiac and the hard, small one as a counterpotion for either sex. Dioscorides also suggests wild lettuce to cool off when the cot gets too hot.

It is not known how all the classical terms—*serapias, kynosorchis, orchishircina, eruthronion,* and *trifolium,* which Dioscorides says has roots as big as apples—correspond to the modern names of the dozens of eligible species that grow in the Mediterranean area. Their use lived on into modern times. The *Ars Magica* of Athanasius Kircher tells how to use the roots and claims, "They'll make an old fellow of sixty-five cut a caper like a Dancing Master." The English made an electuary of their dogstones (*Orchis mascula*) boiled in muscatel with chestnuts (previously soaked in the wine), pistachios, pine nuts, cubeb peppers, cinnamon, rocket seed, and sugar. Dogstones appeared in witches' potions for love and conception. Even the related American lady's slipper of New England was supposedly put to the same use.

Perhaps the most potent species were lost, or perhaps the roots' "powers" diminished as the spirit of rationalism gradually replaced magical ideas, until they became a mere restorative, a source of concentrated nutrition. The name satyrion was gradually replaced by salep, borrowed from the Arabic *sahlab,* from *khusa al-thalab,* "testicles for the fox."

Salep became immensely popular in England until replaced by coffee and soon afterward by tea, but the famous Salopian Shop in Fleet Street enjoyed a lively business until the mid nineteenth century. Salep was often carried on ships as reserve food in case supplies ran out. An ounce of the powder in two quarts of water was enough to keep a sailor in working order until landfall. Some doctors prescribed the drink as a weight-gaining tonic, and salep is still a popular beverage in Turkey.

Orchis roots' properties seem almost entirely due to bassorin, a starchlike substance that makes up half their weight. So concentrated is this mucilage that one part powdered salep to fifteen parts water is enough to make a jelly. To make a demulcent tea, the powder is first mixed evenly in ten parts water, then further diluted with ninety parts water and boiled. Milk may be substituted for part or all of the water. Salep also contains about 5 percent proteinaceous material and useful amounts of calcium, potassium, and phosphorus.

The orchid family is large and varied, so it is quite possible that the ones the Greeks and Romans used have been forgotten or used to extinction, leaving us only with this starchoid. Or it may simply be that what to us is a trifling effect made more of an impression on people less used to continual stimulation. Circumstantial evidence for the former idea may be found in the fact that the Chinese have for millennia used several orchids in prosaic ways, as mild restoratives, but in Africa the Zulus chewed the root of *Lissochilus arenarius* and the stem of *Ansellia gigantea* as potent aphrodisiacs. In any case, couples might well consider taking a bite out of the corsage before pinning it to the lady's dress.

# 🌼 *Saw Palmetto Berries* 🌼

ALSO known as sabal or fan palm, *Serenoa serrulata* or *S. repens* grows in dense stands of scrub within one to five miles of the Atlantic shore from South Carolina to Florida. The sweet reddish brown or purple berries look like dark olives, ripe from October to December. For many decades they have been known to herbalists as one of the most fortifying foods for regaining strength after wasting illnesses. They help build up glandular and muscular tissue and can be used by both overweight and underweight people to help normalize their weight. They have been used with some success to reverse atrophy of the testes and increase sperm production. It has also been claimed that long-term use can enlarge underdeveloped breasts. Their effectiveness is greatly increased when combined with damiana. They are one of the safest and most generally beneficial of all aphrodisiacs. If available, fresh berries are best, a dozen or more per day. The same number of dried ones may be eaten as is, reconstituted with water, or powdered and brewed as a tea.

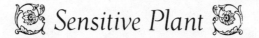 *Sensitive Plant*

SOME tribes of the Amazon basin soak leaves of the *Mimosa pudica* (known here as the houseplant curio touch-me-not or sensitive plant) in juice squeezed from the root. They then apply the leaves to their breasts or the soles of their feet, saying the practice gives them more orgasms and stamina.

Alkaloids can certainly be absorbed this way. Dr. Albert Hoffman discovered the effects of LSD 25 by accidentally absorbing a little through his fingers. Shamans of Old and New Worlds rubbed flying ointments (salves that induce levitation or at least the feeling of flight) on their heads and genitals, and some Arabs and Indians still put powdered henna on their feet, fingers, and temples as a medicine for impotence or premature ejaculation. In the case of the mimosa, however, the plant is known to contain psychedelic tryptamines, but none of them is noted for making plants or people more sensual.

*Mimosa pudica* also seems to be used by certain Peruvian tribes under the name *pencácuc,* "being bashful." They also use the root, but ingest it by mouth. They say the plant grows in male

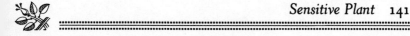

and female forms, that the male incites lust and the female is the antidote.

# 🌀 Vanilla 🌀

THE fermented, unripe fruit of this tropical climbing orchid was one of Madame du Barry's favorite aromatics for erecting her king. Seventeenth-century Mexican physicians used the pods in a digestive cordial, and their mild, stimulating effect on the brain and motor nerves must certainly have been noticed by the Mexican Indians, who added them to their cacao drinks. This happy liaison has persisted ever since.

The active compound seems to be the crystalline aromatic vanillin. Adam Gottlieb suggests that vanilla's uncertain aphrodisiac effect may be a urethral irritation, since vanilla workers often develop inflammation of the hands. The stimulant dose is more than is normally used for flavoring, but because of the probable irritant action, no more than one or two "beans" should be used, and prolonged use is ill-advised. A homemade extract can be made by steeping a pod or two in a pint of brandy for a week or two.

# 🌀 The Plants That 🌀 Time Forgot

EVERY agricultural people derives their beginning from the main food crop, which originally was, they say, their main deity-ancestor, who died and became the first plant of the crop. Plants used in ritual often have a god at their root, too. Many such herbs are no longer known today, but the tales told of them remain to provide employment for scholars. Like the dry-cell battery (known to the Parthian goldsmiths of old Baghdad) and the electrostatic generator (one can be made by following the Biblical directions for the Hebrew Ark of the Covenant), some lost ancient secrets have been rediscovered. The Vedic plant-god Soma has been conclusively identified by R. Gordon Wasson and others as the *Amanita muscaria* mushroom. Like the Sybaritic books of Hemitheon and most of the poetry of Sappho, other legendary plants are permanent casualties of progress. Many of them, real or fabulous, were aphrodisiacs.

On his return from a harrowing trek to the Garden of the Gods, worn-out King Gilgamesh of Erech found pity in the eyes of Utnapishtim the Far Away. To restore the mortal's vigor, spent in quest of his dead friend Enkidu's soul, Utnapishtim revealed a mystery of the gods: "There is a plant that grows under the water; it has a prickle like a thorn, like a rose; it will wound your hands, but if you succeed in taking it, then your hands will hold that which restores his lost youth to a man."

Gilgamesh tied rocks to his feet and jumped in. He found the plant, cut loose the stones, and surfaced, resolved to call it the-old-men-are-young-again and revitalize all the men of his city before using it for himself. But as Gilgamesh took a swim to relax after a day's journey, a serpent crawled into his bag and ate the herb. Gilgamesh and all the rest of us continued to die while snakes got the power to shed old skins for new.

Equally obscure is *katananke*, or catancy, an herb once one of the major ingredients in Thessalian love potions. Nor will you have an easy time finding the *ban to*, a legendary Chinese "peach" that takes three thousand years to ripen but gives sexual youth and eternal life to those who find it.

We have more of a clue about the Greek *telephilon*. Some have suggested a kind of pepper, but a passage in the third idyll of Theocritus seems to indicate the poppy. A goatherd uses one of the leaves of *telephilon* to find out whether his Amaryllis loves him or loves him not. This coincides with a lovers' custom of putting a poppy leaf over the space between the left thumb and forefinger, then striking it with the right palm. If it ruptured with a loud pop, they were beloved; if not, out of luck.

Botanical sleuths have long been paraphrasing Shakespeare in asking, "What is *silphium*?" We know it was an expensive culinary herb much sought by rich Romans and considered erotically stimulating. We know little else, except that most of it came from Cyrene on the Libyan peninsula, but that the best was said to come from Persia. It may have been asafetida; it may be something found around the house; or it may have been a rare herb used up by Roman gourmets. We may never know.

We are sure never to know the powerful aphrodisiac which the Flemish alchemist Jan Baptista van Helmont said is "found everywhere," because the blockhead never recorded its name. Nor are we likely to find any *charisia*, an otherwise unidentified elixir cited in Johannes Clauder's 1661 doctoral dissertation, *De Philtris*. The word seems to be derived from the Greek *charis*, "grace," from which comes charisma. Was it a plant, god's milk shake, or a symbol of charm?

By far the most famous of these herbs is moly, known today mainly by the expression "holy moly." Hermes, the Greek embodiment of masculine Apollonian sun magic, pulls it out of the ground as an amulet for Odysseus to blast the magic drugs of Circe, who holds him and his men bewitched as pigs. Moly overcomes her charms long enough for the hero to threaten her with his sword and make her promise to do him no evil. It also seems to make her lust after him.

Its flowers are white and its root is black, Homer tells us. Theophrastus and Dioscorides thought it was the wild garlic, now called *Allium moly*, and some commentators call it mandrake, although neither really meets the flower-root qualification. The writer of Epigram 69 of the Latin erotic collection *Priapeia* says moly was Odysseus's mentule itself, ". . . for with a leafy branch that yard could hardly be clad." He doesn't explain why the Greek's root was black, although its "white flowers" would still make sense. Still other authors suggest Syrian rue with its sometimes aphrodelic harmal alkaloids, even though its flowers are white with green stripes. As Homer says, ". . . it is hard for mortals to find it, but the gods can do all things."

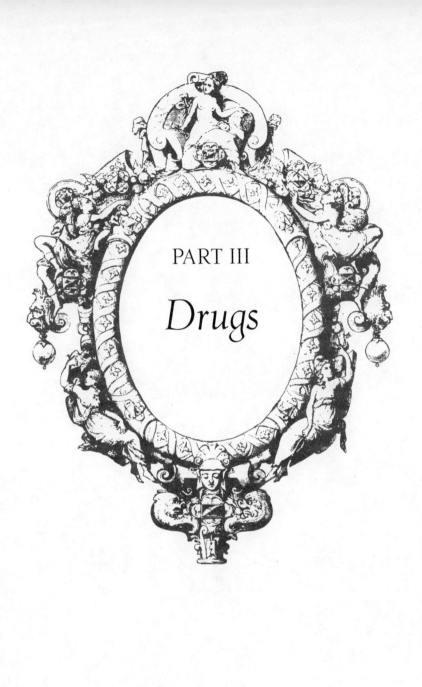

PART III

*Drugs*

*. . . whilst in many places the effect of* Ulysses
*on the reader undoubtedly is somewhat emetic,*
*nowhere does it tend to be an aphrodisiac.*
Ulysses *may, therefore, be admitted*
*into the United States.*
—JUDGE JOHN M. WOOLSEY,
*U.S. v. One Book Called "Ulysses,"*
*5 Federal Supplement* 184 (1933)

ONCE upon a time, a farmer who had been paying less and less attention to his wife sought a doctor's help for his waning sex drive. The doctor examined him, pronounced him basically fit but a bit run-down, and gave him a box of pills, telling him to take one a day and report back in a week. The farmer, a cautious sort, tried a pill on one of his stud bulls. By the end of the first day, the bull had broken out of his stall, thoroughly exhausted every cow in sight, and then knocked down the barn. The farmer got scared and threw the rest of the pills down the well. "Did you drink any of the water?" the sawbones asked worriedly on hearing the tale. "No," admitted the chagrined sodbuster, "we couldn't get the pump handle down."

A medicine with the same kind of power is described in the classic sixteenth-century Chinese novel, *Chin P'ing Mei*. The hero, Hsi-men Ch'ing, obtains his supply from an Indian monk to whom he has shown kindness. The potion is in two parts, a pill that is to be taken with a nip of liquor, and a red powder, a few grains of which are to be dropped into the "horse eye" of the penis just before intercourse.

When Hsi-men first tried it, his penis stood as awesomely erect as a gladiator; ". . . the head swelled and its cyclops eye opened wide; the transverse veins were easily seen; its color was livid as liver; it was nearly seven fingers long and much thicker than usual! Hsi-men was highly pleased. . . . The woman sitting nude on his knees took his penis in her hand and said, 'So this is why you wished to drink spirits.'" Of course, although the pills and powder crop up dozens of times throughout the book, nowhere is their composition so much as hinted at, and we are left holding the legendary bag.

If any such remedy has ever been found, its secret has been well kept. Still, belief dies hard. If many wondrous aphrodisiacs of remote tribes have proven disappointing, some are indirectly worthwhile and others are uninvestigated. If instant elixirs have so far eluded us, hormone therapy has aided many cases of impotence and frigidity. Some scientists confidently predict the first direct, fast-acting aphrodisiac by the year 2000.

Meanwhile, there are easily available drugs that people use to put more flip in their zippers. Alcohol is the most popular, but whether it's the worst because it's legal or legal because it's the worst we'll let the historians of Prohibition decide.

There are always some who turn to heroin, barbiturates, excess holiness, and other depressants as a way of evading their sexuality. But most people who combine drugs and sex do so to increase sensitivity, dissipate the worries of the "real" world ("Reality is for people who can't face drugs," as one wag put it), or free the body-mind from shyness, tension, fear.

A certain Catherine M., contributor to a recent *Oui* magazine reader forum, described the new joy she found in fellatio by way of mescaline: She gave her lover unprecedentedly good head for literally two hours. "It was so smooth and tasty . . . that I could've gone on forever. I was so into it that I thought . . . I was permanently placed in that dream—a cock-sucking machine that had feelings. I was also so into it that it took a few seconds to register the fact that, much to my very stoned boyfriend's surprise, he'd come in my mouth and his come was dribbling down my chin. That made us break into guffaws again, and I think we finally passed out laughing."

A wide variety of chemicals are taken with a common urge—to recover an inno-sense that people feel has been denied or stolen from them. Everyone wants a few hours in the golden age, that mythological era of prehistory or childhood when the body was as free as the sun, with no shadow falling between the emotion and the response, the desire and the spasm. The idea behind the aphrodisiac search is the same as the idea behind several Western heresies and various schools of Hinduism, Islam, and Buddhism—screwing can be divine union, a springboard to satori.

Sexual energy is not limited to the genitals, but diffuses throughout the body like perfume. Several drugs, notably cannabis and the psychedelics, enhance whole-body appreciation of arousal. Call it soul, libido, aura, orgone diffusion, or astral vibrations, sex drugs are taken to spread the energy around, make love less goal oriented, slow down and let the potential build. It's a way of enhancing the physical through the spiritual. For most of these explorers, the search is instinctive. They're unlikely to say much more than, "I get a charge out of it."

Sexy molecules tend to undo instinct suppression. When chemists finally close in on the ultimate aphrodisiac, it may shake things up. Perhaps a vitalizing whiff of sexual wisdom will course through the body politic. Perhaps we'll see a cycle in which sex is promoted as the only leisure activity by something like Huxley's soma, added as a status quo preservative to food and drink. A few decades from now, *anti*aphrodisiacs may be smuggled in diplomatic pouches and sold in washrooms. In any case, it's clear that natives of the future will have more to choose from in the way of erotic stimulants.

Thirty years ago human hormones seemed like the fail-safe potion. Discovery of testosterone's role in arousal raised hopes of intensifying the effects of such sterone-containing plants as sarsaparilla, the *Butea superba* tuber of Thailand, and the *barbasco*, or wild yam, of Latin America (*Dioscorea* genus).

The promise has not been fulfilled. Hormone chemistry is too complex to manipulate externally in most cases. Testosterone shots or pills can bring on delayed sexual maturation or fill in for flagging gonads, but they yield no reliable aphrodisia in healthy people and may even have the opposite result. Synthetic androgens (anabolic steroids) like methandrostenolone may increase desire as well as build muscles, but they often seriously disrupt the body's endocrine balance and pose a cancer threat.

We don't even know whether the androgens work the same way in men and women. Males generally have ten times as much testosterone as females, while women secrete more antrostenedione; both sexes produce equal amounts of dihydroepiandrosterone. The action of estrogen as a sexual damper may also be different in men and women. Thyroid and adrenal hormones play their part, and the whole orchestra is conducted by the anterior pituitary gland and the ancient brain area called the hypothalamus.

A feedback loop of nerves and blood vessels between the two organs controls the flow of pituitary hormones. FSH (follicle stimulating hormone) provokes growth of the egg follicle on the ovary and secretion of estrogen in the first part of a woman's cycle. As the egg matures, the pituitary's LH (luteinizing hormone) turns the follicle into a corpus luteum (yellow body) that secretes the pregnancy-preparing hormone progestin, which overshadows estrogen in the woman's other fortnight. Neither of the ovarian hormones has a decisive influence on desire; as many women report their peak sensuality in one phase as in the other.

The same pituitary hormones are known by different names in men because they perform different functions. FSH equals spermatogenic hormone. LH is called ICSH (interstitial cell stimulating hormone) because it goads the interstitial (Leydig) cells in the testes (and adrenal cortices of both sexes) to secrete desire-producing androgens. Pituitary concentrates can often aid those in whom the gland functions poorly, but the nitty-gritty of its work is still poorly understood, and we have no aphrodisiac that will go directly from the mouth (or nose) to trip an erotic reaction in the head.

Still, the search for the brain-key goes on, led by tantalizing hints that have never been more numerous. Experiments in which a microscopic tubule (cannula) is implanted in an animal's brain seem to have located an "erotic funnel" at the junction between the front hypothalamus and preoptic region in the limbic system (old cortex), through which any sensory or motor impulse must pass before it can elicit a sexual response.

Its discovery has given new language to the old "left-handed" path of spiritual enlightenment (through sexual prolongation), common to Taoist, Tantric, and Gnostic systems of sex magic. Most of the surviving literature on these practices makes the man into a sort of psychic succubus, for whom the woman exists only to nourish. But it now makes more sense to see the rites as a way for both sexes to awaken the intuitive, inward focusing (left-handed) right hemisphere of the brain, using it to get beyond the left hemisphere's logicality, directing awareness to the base of erotic feeling in the preconscious old brain by using the tremendous energy yield of hours-long lovemaking—a sort of sexual meditation.

The brain's erotic gateway also opens the road to more material aphrodisiacs. A droplet of estrogen at the portal induces mating in female rats. ACTH (adrenocorticotropic hormone, a pituitary humor that gets the adrenals to make cortisone) also works as an aphrodisiac when implanted in rodent brains. Scientists studying endorphins (morphine-like compounds made by the body) have found that they block sexual desire, while opiate antagonists like naloxone enhance it, at least in rats. And several compounds tested on humans, while not exactly elixirs, at least brighten the lust horizon.

One of the things that happens to the brain as it gets older is a degeneration of nerve pathways that use the neurotransmitters dopamine, epinephrine, and norepinephrine—the catecholamines, which are normally made in our bodies from 1–dopa (dihydroxyphenylalanine), a precursor in turn made from the amino acid tyrosine in our diet. These electrochemical pathways drive all the hormone-balancing work of the pituitary gland. As these catecholamine pathways decay, they are slowly replaced by others using a different transmitter, serotonin.

In cases of extreme dopamine loss (Parkinson's disease), an external source of the precursor, levadopa, can for a time restore the function. The dramatic return of sexual desire in patients was at first hailed as the sign of the aphrodisiac, but an endless list of side effects pertains, and no rushes of desire occur from it in youthful animals or humans.

PCPA (parachlorophenylalanine) was tested after researchers at the National Heart Institute tried it on a woman with bowel cancer. She got permission for her husband to stay at the hospital because "she was trying to grab everybody." Dr. Allesandro Tagliamonte studied the substance further on rats and found "hypersexual aggression," lasting for several hours and ending with "all the animals in one cage attempting to mount each other at the same time."

PCPA seems to work by inhibiting the production of serotonin, antagonizing the sexual antagonist, as it were. But it too has an emerging list of problems. In humans it seems to take several days for any effect to show, then several days to wear off, during which time slecp is impossible and exhaustion inevitable. This property may have given birth to the rumor of a mythical three-day aphrodisiac called "steam" a few years ago.

Dr. Joseph Meites of Michigan State University Medical School has worked with both of these compounds. He and his colleagues have succeeded in rejuvenating aged female rats whose estrous cycles have stopped, the effect proven by pregnancy. No live young have been born yet, because the long-unused womb is subject to infection. Dr. Meites points out that the ovaries of old rats can be reactivated, but those of old humans cannot, because the ovaries shrink up like an appendix so that new hormones have no reverse effect. Male rats are much closer to humans in that the decrease in sperm and hormone production seems to be a reversible process.

One of the most promising of the dopaminergic helpers is part of the same complex of drugs made by the ergot rye fungus that gave us LSD. Bromergocryptine, or simply bromocryptine, has been available by prescription in West Germany and Switzerland for several years. In experiments at the University of Siena, Italy, scientists found the drug restored menstruation in all eleven women tested, whose cycles had stopped for as long as twelve years. In other tests in Sweden and Holland, sexual desire awoke in many "frigid" women. In some who "never had erotic feelings in their entire lives, bromocryptine led to normal sexual activity," concluded Dr. Andrea Genazzini.

The surprising thing is that there have been no adverse effects noted so far. In late 1978 bromocryptine was approved by the U.S. Food and Drug Administration for prescription use in cases of galactorrhea amenorrhea. This is a condition, usually postpartum, in which milk flow never stops and menstruation never restarts. By fortifying the dopamine pathways, bromocryptine inhibits the milk-secreting hormone prolactin and stimulates production of the gonadotropic hormones.

Still other molecules, like antiserotonergic ergot derivative methysergide, will be checked out in coming years. But there is no evidence that any of them have much effect on healthy people. Two things—fear and orgasm—have been produced in animals by direct electrical stimulation of the appropriate parts of the brain. Maybe the true aphrodisiac is somewhere we'd hardly thought of looking—in the socket.

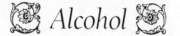

# Alcohol

*If I take one drink, I can't feel it;*
*If I take two drinks, I can feel it;*
*If I take three drinks, anyone can feel it.*
—ANONYMOUS

OUR ancestors discovered alcohol long before they invented writing, so all we can say about its origin is that it has been part of sacred and secular rituals for thousands of years. Ethyl alcohol was probably not the first mind-changing drug humans noticed, but it is one of the easiest to prepare and has been the most common social lubricant in nearly every known culture. No other substance flows so ubiquitously through our myth and history. Probably no other has given us so much pleasure and so much trouble.

Ethyl ($CH_3CH_2OH$) alcohol's first definite appearance is in the depiction of a brewery on an Egyptian tomb about 3700 B.C. Words for beer and must (fermenting grape juice) occur before 3000 B.C. in Mesopotamia, where beer was brewed in the temples. The mythical flood-hero of later Babylonians turns up as Noah in the Bible, who settled as a vintner on Ararat after the Big Wash. Noah's love of the bubbly was so great that it was later used to justify Israel's destruction of the peoples of Canaan. The Canaanites were descended from Ham, Noah's youngest son, whom he cursed for telling his brothers that their father was dead-drunk and nude in his tent.

Grapes grew wild throughout the Caspian–Caucasus–Near Eastern region, so wild in fact, that when the Israelite spies returned from their reconnaissance of the Promised Land, they brought back *one bunch* on a staff between two men. Fermentation, of course, must have been noticed thousands of years before that, the first time someone ate a mess of overripe grapes (or berries or other fruit or wet grain or honey) fermenting in the summer sun. This discovery must have been made many times throughout the world, for the Spaniards found American Indians drinking a corn beer called *chicha*; Dr. Livingstone found the Central Africans sipping palm wine; and nearly every aboriginal group except the Eskimos have their own native booze.

The Persians, in explaining its discovery, tell the tale of King Jamshid, who loved grapes so much that he stored the excess of a bountiful harvest in jars in the palace cellar. Sending for them months later, he was dismayed to find they had disintegrated into a smelly liquid and sent them back labeled POISON. Soon thereafter, a love-crossed woman of the court, contemplating suicide, drank some of the stuff to end her misery and was surprised to find her misery gone but herself still there. After Jamshid put her story to the proof, he named the beverage *zeher-e-kush* ("poison of delight") and decreed part of each harvest should be spoiled thus.

At first it was magic, of course; a new spirit was worshiped, which soon spread from temple and palace to hut and slave quarters, until the first-dynasty Babylonian king Hammurabi felt the need to safeguard his subjects' health by writing quality standards for Babylonian taverns into his famous code of laws. Lest we think the sage ancients had any less of a problem with the drug, nearly every society has been violently pro and con, and most have tried to prohibit it. From the very beginning, literature shows the same variety of reaction, from giddiness and good dirty fun to moroseness to violence to stupor, and the same danger of alcoholism to too large a minority. Ethyl has always kept soldiers happy (the Egyptian infantryman got a quart of wine or beer a day). And the Persians hollered the same boast we often hear today: "We Persians can drink deeper than anybody without seeming half so drunk" (usually delivered pompously in that improbable Leaning-Tower-of-Pisa stance that gives it all away).

Wine flowed through the veins of Osiris, then Dionysus, then Bacchus. Bacchus's sparkling blood flowed out the veins of Jesus who, like these predecessor gods, died to give the world a rejuvenating elixir—the wine he made at the Cana wedding for his first miracle. Long before that, Homeric sailors were pouring libations to their gods. That burning antifreeze, warmth against sea winds and courage for the conquest, has been on every ship since. When the S.S. *Constitution* sailed her maiden voyage, for example, she set out with 79,400 gallons of rum and 48,600 of water for her crew of 475. En route she picked up another 172,600 gallons of assorted spirits, then docked six months later, empty but for the untouched stagnant water.

As an aphrodisiac, alcohol is unique. It is by far the worst, but still the most popular, the universally proverbial prelude to seduction. And yet any man who has *limped* through a bout of drunken impotence will swear to ethyl's antagonism to amour.

In ancient times the servants customarily tied flowers and sweet herbs around guests' heads to ward off wine's ill effects. Dutch sexologist Theodor Hendrik van de Velde recommended it only as far as a "mild degree of that slightly merry and carefree intoxication which is far from drunkenness," and cautioned that drink in the cause of Venus should always be accompanied with food to slow down absorption. Shakespeare put the case plainly when he had the porter tell Macduff (*Macbeth*, Act II, Scene 3) what three things drink provokes: "Marry, sir, nose-painting, sleep, and urine. Lechery, sir, it provokes, and unprovokes: it provokes the desire, but it takes away the performance . . . it makes him stand to, and not stand to. . . ." As Masters and Johnson would say, it stimulates arousal but hinders plateau and orgasm. This is one reason why Bacchus was always portrayed as a beardless eunuch.

Once more an unknown rhymster put it most succinctly:

> *There was a young man name Hughes*
> *Who swore off all kinds of booze.*
> *He said, "When I'm muddled*
> *My senses get fuddled,*
> *And I pass up too many screws."*

Usually classed as a central nervous system depressant, alcohol seems to anesthetize the nerves, starting with the most recent, logical part of the brain, the cerebral cortex. Thus it hits us first where the social restrictions and inhibitions lie, but it soon goes on to affect the rest of the nervous system. Like many other drugs, it is vaguely said to provoke a high by dissolving the rigid ego a bit, liberating thoughts and feelings usually kept in Freud's locked attic. No one knows exactly how this works, but the alcohol high is so full of "static"—so soon overshadowed by the physical unpleasantness—that pharmacologists call it a "paradoxical intoxication."

Of course, individual responses vary widely. Some get staggering drunk or belligerent or suicidal on one or two; others can carry on almost normally, glass after glass, all night long. In general, alcohol produces incoordination which, contrary to popular myth, is not helped by practicing a lot while drunk. Moreover, many drinkers remain unaware of this clumsiness, even in bed.

Folklore and statistics abound, from Aristotle's account of Alexander's love life atrophied by wine to modern studies of alcoholics and their impotence, frigidity, premature senility, and deterioration of the reproductive glands. Beyond this, little is known of the immediate effects of more moderate drinking on human sex life, except that it lowers sperm count and motility and produces structural damage in some sperm that may increase the risk of birth defects.

As usual, we know more about dogs and rats. In them, all forms of "copulatory behavior" are depressed. The male is slower to attain erection and doesn't mount as often; the estrous cycle of females is disrupted. The males do take longer to ejaculate, which might raise some hopes for liquor as a defense against prematurity, but the price of decreased sensitivity makes this a last-ditch cure.

The body burns ethanol in a two-step process, mostly in the liver, which undergoes a drastic change in chemical condition in seconds after alcohol hits it. Alcohol prevents the liver from metabolizing many nutrients, including amino acids, some sugars, fatty acids, glycerol, steroids, and monoamines. It depletes the organ's reserves of vitamin C and thiamine (vitamin $B_1$), a result accentuated by fasting, poor nutrition, or hypothyroidism. Hence alcohol has always been known to be especially destructive to persons in the old medical classification of neurasthenia—thin, undernourished, or nervous.

Many of the alcoholic brews of the past must have been nutritious enough in their other ingredients to offset many of alcohol's deficits. The thick beers and stouts of Elizabethan England, for example, were recently estimated to have had five times as much calcium and magnesium, eight times as much riboflavin (vitamin $B_2$), and ten times as much niacin ($B_3$) as their modern counterparts. And the typical American stein has only half the nutrients of British beer. Recipes for concentrated classical wines—some the Romans made were as thick as jelly—have been lost, and the continuing trend to purification, distillation, and carbonization has diluted grog's food value to little more than alcohol's basic 7 calories per gram.

These readily available calories may be what gives alcohol its aphrodisiac reputation. How drunk you get certainly depends on how fast your body can burn them. Since the idea is to maintain that first flush of bibulous stimulation as long as possible, the obvious stratagem is to drink alcohol only as fast as the body can metabolize it. The average is .6 to .75 ounce per hour. A 150-pound person of average tolerance can absorb about half a shot (half a glass of wine or a half-pint of beer) per hour without feeling it. Once this goes up to one shot per hour, blood alcohol levels build up over .05 percent and first the cortex, then (at .10 percent) the rest of the body, is affected. The ancient art of watering the wine, one of the host's main duties, developed to regulate intake and allow guests to satisfy a thirst—but still last all night.

Alcohol also makes the drinker piss a lot. Stimulation of urine flow is sometimes misinterpreted as excitation of the associated sexual organs, as in the use of Spanish fly, but this cannot really be called aphrodisia. The flow results not only from the drink itself, at least half of which is usually water, but from ethanol's impairment of secretion of the body's antidiuretic hormone, which normally keeps urine from passing too quickly through the kidneys before they can filter efficiently.

When Ogden Nash, pointing the way to a woman's heart, quipped, "Candy is dandy, but liquor is quicker," he may have been hit by pharmacological prescience. Alcohol does seem to have effects on women that it does not on men. It suppresses the release of oxytocin, a reproductive hormone secreted in the posterior pituitary and needed for contracting the uterus during labor. Lack of oxytocin also prevents secretion of milk for the baby afterward. In fact, two 1967 medical studies found that liquor effectively delayed birth when labor began prematurely, usually in tiny amounts of 30 milliliters (about one ounce or two-thirds jigger) of cognac, three times a day.

On the more speculative side, there is the result of one experiment with chickens, in which roosters started behaving like mother hens to the new chicks they usually attack. Joseph K. Kovach of the Menninger Foundation found that when left alone with new-hatched chicks for five days, sober roosters either let them die of exposure or stomped and pecked them to death. But all five of the drunken cocks sheltered the young ones at night. Two gradually reverted to normal, but three defended the youngsters against the others and even started clucking like hens when sobriety returned.

This is, of course, tenuous evidence to propose a unique or stronger effect of alcohol on women than on men, but it receives a little support in the Playboy-Research Guild survey, *Sexual Behavior in the 1970s*. Interviewers found that 36 percent of women said alcohol makes sex more pleasant, compared to 30 percent of the men. And 27 percent of the males said it lessened enjoyment, but only 12 percent of the females agreed.

Alcohol may help the pathologically shy, whom A. F. Niemoller describes as "the timid soul who, while feeling the prick of the flesh, still starts and flushes at the proximity of a bed and the necessity of disrobement." But the first instance of drunken inability is likely to make this sort more bashful still.

Statistical correlation of inebriation with aggressive acts is too strong to ignore and, in men filled with repressed hatred of women, alcohol facilitates release in the form of rape. The literature of bygone cultures, where a sober man was hardly called a man, continually flirts with sanctioned sexual violence, while the cult of chastity in effect made force essential to copulation.

The role of alcohol in this kind of situation was recently confirmed by an experiment that showed that, when drunk, men respond less to whimsical humor and more to aggressive humor based on cruelty. Granted that most men who drink don't end up as rapists, the tendency in this direction can no more qualify as aphrodisia than the urinary stimulation can. The question remains: Why would anyone want to take an anesthetic before making love?

The answer, I feel, is connected to patriarchal Western society's profound fear of sex in general and women in particular. This fear goes back at least as far as dualistic philosophy's assignment of the body to Hell, the spirit to Heaven. It is odd that the Church, while condemning drunkenness, preserved the Roman vineyards as the Empire collapsed—and not only for the paltry needs of the sacrament. Monasteries were usually centers of wine making and many become Europe's first distilleries. Consciously or not, the holy fathers chose to produce the most harmful common drug, known *even in ancient times* to cause bodily damage, and one that carried the built-in retribution of a hangover, along with the likelihood of drunken sins to foster the guilt that invited further mortification of the flesh.

As the West's only socially sanctioned intoxicant before caffeine and nicotine, alcohol was a natural choice for men who valued aggression and conquest above the "weaker" virtues. This is not to say that wine made ravenous beasts out of Omar Khayyám, Socrates, and many other gentle banqueteers, for ultimately it is the individual who determines the effects of the drug, not vice versa. We must conclude that alcohol is the most popular aphrodisiac only by default, for those who feel they must take *something* when nothing else is handy.

But other things can be dissolved *in alc*ohol. The second most universal solvent, alcohol stores the essences of herbs, including the aphrodisiacs. Jamaicans soak *ganja* (cannabis) in bottles of rum; Strega and Benedictine and Chartreuse each have their legends and secret formulas.

The fin-de-siècle floating drunk of absinthe can be approximated by soaking one to two tablespoons of wormwood (*Artemisia absinthium*) in a bottle of Pernod or other anisette liqueur, perhaps diluted with a little neat spirits, as real absinthe was 136 proof. Soak the herb for two days or more, then filter. Note that, although the herb is legal, the drink is not, and large quantities are probably mildly toxic, though little is known for sure on this point.

You can try the seventeenth-century favorite, Fortuna Veneris. Gather two handfuls of the biggest, sourest-smelling pismires (ants) you can find. Steep them in a gallon of brandy, then distill the mixture three times "till all be dry." Pour off the oil from the top of the fluid, then add cinnamon for flavor. This potion is supposed to instill battle courage as well as "wonderfully irritate them that are slothful to venery." The formic acid from the ants, a caustic end product of wood-alcohol poisoning, and responsible for the sting of nettles, certainly would irritate!

The brew usually retains much of the character of its source. Mead, perhaps the oldest drink of all, is almost as famous in the bedroom as honey. The various honey ales and wines were drunk in huge quantities throughout Europe until they were displaced by the beer industry.

Since the time of the Greeks or before, wine has served as the base for many an elixir. Among the most famous is *hippocras*, beloved of the Romans and revived in Europe by Paracelsus and François Villon. The classic recipe calls for:

*One ounce each crushed cinnamon and ginger, ⅓ ounce cloves and vanilla pods, and 2¼ pounds raw sugar, all steeped in a bottle of red Burgundy for five days. This mixture is then strained through a cloth and poured through a funnel containing a sachet of 1½ grains ambergris, ⅓ grain pure musk, and $^1/_7$ ounce rock candy. An ounce of the result is then added to whatever wine is in the glass.*

I have been unable to form definite conclusions about this potion, for lack of ambergris, but musk taken internally brings a strange warmth to the skin and an unctuous sweet luxury to the lips.

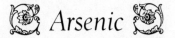

# Arsenic

THE recurrent use of poisons as love potions bears out the ancient theme that death is a grand form of orgasm. Use of arsenic to explore this boundary is probably very old, for the Greek word for the semimetallic element, *arsenikon*, comes directly from the adjective *arsenikos*, meaning masculine.

Arsenic's chemical similarity to phosphorus allows it to readily replace this essential mineral in the body's nerves and glands, leading first to mild vasodilatation and stimulation. In larger doses blood pressure falls and shock, kidney damage, headache, nausea, and diarrhea all set in. Swelling from capillary damage at low doses may have been misinterpreted as a tonic effect.

The history of medicine discloses many experimental arsenicals, often including quinine, iron, and nux vomica for good measure, all now discarded. Arsenic's garlic smell was often just barely noticeable in cattle feed, to which it was long added to boost the growth rate before the advent of diethylstilbestrol. In like manner, arsenic patent medicines were sold to women as breast developers and complexion enhancers. The element probably had some effect in external use for the same reason that it preserves parchment, paper, or hunting trophies—it kills any bacteria or molds that try to attack the treated material.

An arsenic-eating fad swept through parts of Europe in the mid-1860s; at least there was a big ballyhoo in the press over it, but few reports of fatalities. Tyrolean peasants from the middle Styria district of Austria were reported to eat up to 6 grains of pure white arsenic on their daily bread without harm. An 1865 issue of the Edinburgh Medical Journal summarized the phenomenon, but it soon vanished from the public eye, leaving arsenic once more to fumigators and kindly little spinsters in old lace sipping elderberry wine.

# 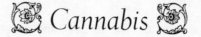 *Cannabis*

*Every man and every woman is a star.*
—the goddess Nuit through
Aleister Crowley,
*The Book of the Law*

IT WAS fresh, nectarous Lebanese, blonde as the summer sun, and being in the first flush of a long love affair, we had only one idea about how to try it out. The high was like a strong wind, gusting to forty knots, with none of that humid lethargy of some hash, and we fell to our double feast without so much as a napkin. After a long overture, we were in the opening passages of the pas de deux when our individual consciousnesses were disconnected by a force from above, or within, or elsewhere, and our bodies merged into the reunited metasexual being that Aristophanes named our ancestor. Our single body snapped back and forth like a jackhammer, pleasuring itself with an industrial speed and precision far beyond our conscious will and, we would have thought, beyond the capacities of mere protoplasm. I suppose the machine ran in overdrive for about a half hour of clock time before it blew its fuses in a blinding blue-white shower of sparks. We returned to our usual selves gasping, wondering why we couldn't smell ozone.

If only there were a substance that could infallibly bring that fragile ecstasy; yet no more than fresh air and excitement can do the same about as often. We were left closer to our instincts. Like about half of the fifteen to thirty million American pot users, we found that cannabis has few equals as a safe but capricious erotic catalyst.

To get the bad news over with early, let us note that grass may have some of the same adverse health effects that tobacco has, since its smoke contains 20 percent more tars per gram than tobacco. But so much careless research was hawked in the early 1970s to scare people away from the pot menace that any study which shows real dangers now inevitably seems like a cry of wolf to other scientists and newsmen. I find it hard to believe that one kind of hot smoke causes cancer while another (smoked in smaller quantities but even hotter and inhaled more deeply) is totally harmless. I suspect that propagandists, for whatever cause, always shield our eyes from the full glare of actuality. Still, even heavy pot smoking is demonstrably one of the least dangerous habits available.

Claims have been prematurely made that marijuana damages chromosomes, causes breast development in males, lowers testosterone levels and decreases sperm count, leads to loss of sex drive and the will to succeed, weakens the immune response to disease and causes brain damage. Not one has been confirmed. One famous flap resulted when the usually reliable medical journal *Lancet* said in an editorial that pot literally causes the brain to wither away. Most news media failed to read some of the fine print of the report itself to find that the conclusion was based on only ten test subjects, most of whom had many other drug habits and/or a history of head injury and mental illness.

An enormous amount of research (we have studied marijuana more than any other drug in the world) has laid these fears to rest. Surveys of human smokers—including many in Jamaica and Costa Rica who inhale more ganja in a week than most Americans do in their lives—have failed to show *any* health problems definitely caused or aggravated by cannabis use. If the plant has a detrimental effect on sexual function, then it is odd that surveys in the United States have shown that marijuana smokers average 60 to 80 percent *more* sexual activity than nonsmokers—even though this can be partly explained by the greater lust for experience that led the one group to try an illegal pleasure in the first place.

Norman Mailer was one of the first to write about marijuana's effects on lovemaking, and his comments agree well with what so many others found years later: "It gets into parts of me that nothing else can reach; it relaxes tensions only sex can approach—and sex is invariably truer with pot. You can learn to use your body better. The same move you make every day takes on more meaning."

Naturally, there are dissenters. Some people find that sex feels worse when they're stoned. Summing up this side, Gay Talese wrote: "Nothing will thwart performance more decisively than being stoned, because you're mellowed out and become slovenly." Another thing that thwarts performance is performance worries, and they can be frightfully magnified by marijuana.

According to Dr. Erich Goode's 1969 questionnaire survey for the *Evergreen Review* ("Marijuana and Sex," no. 55 [1969], p. 19) only 5 percent of users reported a negative sexual effect; 51 percent said it had no definite result or depended on the mood, while 44 percent said the weed invariably turned their thought bedward. That the pleasures of cannabis must be learned was shown in that only 44 percent of the "infrequent" smokers said they enjoyed sex more while high, while 77 percent of "frequent" users did.

A joint or a pipe will probably stay the favorite means of ingestion for a long time; the euphoria comes quickly and the dose is easily regulated. Those who can find it will savor the powerful, almost lysergic rush of purified hash oil, vaporized and inhaled from little glass pipes. But for sustained (though more unpredictable) ecstasy combined with a taste treat, nothing tops the hashish confection usually called *majoon*, common from Morocco to India but lamentably rare here because of the high cost of importation. I will allow Gautier, Ludlow, and Baudelaire to describe its delights and terrors; to experience them, the following Moroccan recipe is a good start:

> Thoroughly toast about ½ ounce cleaned marijuana (twigs and seeds removed) in a heavy skillet over a slow fire. Stir it constantly until it reaches a golden brown without burning. About 3–7 grams powdered hashish or ½–1 gram hash oil may be substituted without pre-cooking. If using toasted grass, pound it fine in a mortar and pestle.
>
> Mix the main ingredient with 1 cup finely chopped dates, ½ cup chopped raisins, 1 cup ground almonds and walnuts (or any other combination of nuts), 1 cup finely chopped figs, 1 teaspoon ground fresh ginger, 1 teaspoon ground cinnamon, 1 whole grated nutmeg, 1 tablespoon ground aniseed, and ½ cup honey. Mix and cook together with ½ cup water until the mass is softened and the water absorbed or evaporated. Melt 2 tablespoons butter or ghee over a low flame and add the majoon. Cook a few minutes, cool, and stir in ¼ cup or less orange-flower water (optional), and store in an airtight jar.

A level tablespoon per person is a good dose to start with. It may not be enough, but too much can be scary and demoralizing, although not physically dangerous. Increase the amount slowly in subsequent voyages, if necessary. When eaten, cannabis can be a very potent psychedelic, so if you plan to make love, you will not want to overdo it, at least when the drug is still new to you. A cup of hot mint tea provides traditional atmosphere and also aids absorption.

Many people have tried to explain why cannabis so often heightens the sexual experience. The consensus is that it amplifies the impact of our senses—especially the tactile—on the brain, and helps release the mind from guilt or shyness, leading to better fantasies; the relaxed sense of time (or timelessness) provides the ideal setting to act them out.

Perhaps the archenemy of marijuana, former U.S. Commissioner of Narcotics Harry J. Anslinger, said it best: "In the earliest stages of intoxication, the will power is destroyed . . . moral barricades are broken down, and often debauchery and sexuality result." A mid-1960s potboiler called *The Mind Benders* (written under the appropriately pustular pseudonym Lance Boyle) tells the tragic tale of "Miriam," who found herself making ecstatic love to "Scott" and actually enjoying it, "even though he was a Negro." The drug made it all right, though: "It wasn't really me there, you see. It was someone else who could do all these things and not suffer any recriminations in the morning."

What it all comes down to, then, is a bit of hocus-pocus, a trance that awakens us from our trance, a hole in unreal reality through which we can grab a piece of our birthright—transubstantiation into living divinities, whose bodies are huge, unmapped erogenous zones with no forbidden territory.

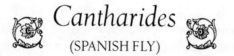

# *Cantharides*
## (SPANISH FLY)

IN MANY parts of Asia, Russia, and southern Europe live beautiful shiny green and gold beetles, up to an inch long with heads shaped like Valentine hearts, giving off an unusual and elusive odor as they gaudily munch on lilac, honeysuckle, elder, ash, and other leaves. Driven by hunger or curiosity, a few hardy souls here and there sampled the bugs and soon found themselves on fire, burning hottest in the crotch and uncontrollably humping every prong or hole in sight. I doubt that many of them recommended the experience, but to others, the sight of a normal person suddenly copulating in a frenzy for days must have seemed awfully attractive. Despite reports of pain, visions of supernatural sex must have kept the legend alive in each generation.

The insect we now call Spanish fly (*Lytta vesicatoria*) has moved in the underworld of the most dramatic love philters of recorded history. From India to Morocco it is added to majoon when desperate lust bribes the cook. In China it was, and perhaps still is, given in a syrup of honey, saffron, cinnamon, nutmeg, cloves, and cubeb pepper. Known to Greeks and Romans as *cantharis*, it was probably the main ingredient in the strongest Roman love cups, although no recipes survive. As in India, the beetle was probably mixed with datura as well, for a truly overwhelming experience and convenient amnesia afterward.

Cantharides found a small but steady market in medieval Arabia and Europe. One of the recipes current then survives in the *Geneanthropeia* of Sinibaldis:

> *Tincture of Spanish fly (½ teaspoon), Spanish lavender (2 tablespoons), spirits of chloroform (1 teaspoon). Dilute with water to 8 ounces and take 2 tablespoons three times a day. [Winged ants were sometimes substituted for the beetles.]*

Elsewhere an occasional risky fling, Spanish fly enjoyed a great vogue among the eighteenth-century French aristocracy. It was made into all kinds of candies and cakes for private affairs, and sold in pills as *pastilles galantes*. Grandval, in his play *The Two Biscuits*, describes the double use of cantharides and opium to counteract each other:

> *One was made of cantharis flies,*
> *Which sickly lovers' strength restores;*
> *In the other ruled the opium pod,*
> *Whose powers make one sleep like a clod.\**

\* Literally "like a clog," wooden shoe.

The later writer of *The Private Life of Louis XV's Mistresses* felt compelled to explain the manic interest in aphrodisiacs thus: "Spanish fly, *diabolini* [Italian for 'devil pastilles'], essence of gillyflowers [cloves], ambergris enemas, etc., are the inventions of our century, in which debility has been incurable without these aids." The Marquis de Sade was one of the beetle sellers' best customers, but was paradoxically proven innocent of giving the drug in chocolate bonbons to guests at one of his private orgies in Marseilles. Retaliating for his sadistic treatment of her daughter, his mother-in-law gave the court enough testimony about his other habits to get him sentenced to death anyway, forcing him to flee to Italy.

Mad William Windom, the so-called King of London's streetwalkers in the mid nineteenth century, continued the upper-class fly tradition by serving a party punch made from a small amount of cantharides, champagne, curaçao, various herbs, soda water, and sugar. But for the most part the French Revolution relegated Spanish fly to locker-room jokes and street-corner fantasies.

There was good reason for neglect. Hearsay had begun to transmit the disasters as well as the bogus ecstasies. Spanish flies killed their countryman, Ferdinand of Castile. Cabrol, a pupil of French court physician Ambroise Paré, recorded a famous case of 1572. A man of Provence, ill with a quartan fever, had been given 1½ ounces of nettles (an irritant itself) and 2 drams of cantharides. Depending on which dram measure was used, this would be 3.5 or 7.8 grams; as little as 1.5 grams can be fatal. He was the victim of satyriasis so painful that ". . . his wife swore to us by her God that he had been astride her, during two nights, eighty-seven times, without thinking it more than ten . . . and even while we were interviewing him, the poor man ejaculated thrice in our presence, embracing the foot of the bed and moving against it as if it were his wife."

This man apparently lived, but others were not so lucky. Another victim, after ramming his wife forty times in one night, was tied up in a wet sheet to keep him from hurting himself; a priest was called to exorcise him, but before he could arrive the man was dead, his cock already gangrenous. A man described by Nicolas Venette, poisoned by a rival whose mistress he'd married, barely survived a night of exhaustion, fever, and bleeding from the penis caused by a mere 2 or 3 grains (130 to 195 milligrams).

In a woman the drug can provoke uterine hemorrhage or abortion if she is pregnant. One of the most famous first-year English law cases is that of the British wholesale pharmacist who gave two young girls some coconut ice spiked with cantharides. They died almost immediately, and today most copies of that volume of cases opens automatically to "The Love Potion That Went Wrong." Sadly, no similar notoriety followed the mid-1950s case of an American coed found dead in a car with the gearshift up her bleeding vagina after having been slipped Spanish fly at a college dance.

The verdict is clear. The supposed erotic effects of Spanish fly are functional excitation without desire or pleasure; they result from its caustic, blistering action on the intestines, urethra, and any other flesh it touches. Other reactions include retching, shock, and purging, enough to take the fun out of any seduction. Susceptibility to the active ingredient, cantharidin, varies. Great pain or death can occur, and the results are not worth the risks of even the *tiniest* doses.

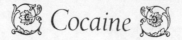 Cocaine

*Chew my 'baccer, spit my juice,*
*Gonna love my baby till it ain't no use*
*An' ho ho, baby, take a whiff on me.*

. . .

*Cocaine for horses an' not for men,*
*Doctors say it'll kill you but they don't say when*
*An' ho ho, baby, take a whiff on me.*
—LEADBELLY

A SHOT of cocaine feels more like an orgasm than anything in the world except an orgasm. A snort is less explosive but is still universally described in terms of the flash and the afterglow. In a laboratory study by George R. Gay and Charles W. Sheppard, ten out of twenty men who had just had an injection got immediate erections, and two of them stayed hard for nearly a day, long after the drug had worn off. Women have been known to come from the rush—no hands, no tools. No wonder that for some of its heavy users cocaine *is* sex even more than it is *for* sex.

Even when contained in the much milder and safer coca leaves from which it comes, cocaine was adored by the Andean Indians, who said "God is a substance." Depending on the dose, it bestows anything from a subtle lift to a rush of energy that feels superhuman. It can be experienced as mental or physical. Sometimes the energy is expressed in a logical flood, flights of ideas, and a loquaciousness that precludes much interest in amour. Sir Arthur Conan Doyle, for example, solved his detective's knottiest problems with it.

Some find the speedup a bit too racelike for love; some mitigate it by combining it with grass. Norman Douglas, for example, found cocaine took him to a Playboy-like "paradise where Venus may be seen, but not touched." But for others the white dust can fuel passion long past the usual limits of endurance. Men can often keep it up and surging for hours, to the point where vaginal secretions run dry and one has to take a lubrication break. Erection can sometimes be maintained even after one or more ejaculations.

On the other side of the coin, after too much coke over the course of a day or a week, the body's energy storehouses are gone and the same sexual phenomena go too far: "control" may reach the point of frustration beyond which orgasm can no longer occur until the body takes a long, slow, painful ride back to equilibrium. Several lovers of male coke dealers have confided that toot tends to displace sex when the supply is too good.

Since cocaine is the best local anesthetic known, a little bit dissolved in cream or lotion is sometimes applied to the glans penis to prevent premature ejaculation or to the glans clitoris to aid long tonguing and fingering when soreness following orgasm would otherwise prevent it. However, because the best (still much cut) bootleg cocaine sells for up to a hundred dollars a gram (twenty dollars an ounce legally for surgery), most people who merely want a desensitizer use lidocaine or Solarcaine.

Unlike too much pot, an overdose of cocaine can be fatal as well as unpleasant. This danger is complicated by wide variations among individuals in their response to the drug and is compounded by the ignorance bred by prohibition and official half-truths.

The average fatal single dose is quoted by doctors as about 1.2 grams, a truly enormous amount that is only approached in rare medical situations. Indeed, nearly all the recorded deaths from cocaine have occurred in hospitals. However, serious toxic reactions can occur among the few people who are allergic to cocaine in amounts as small as 20 milligrams. Warning signs include cold or profuse sweat, pallor, severe anxiety or aggressiveness, and a feeling of heaviness in the limbs. Although these symptoms are so rare as to be almost nonexistent among those who snort the drug rather than shoot it (usually as a flip side to a heroin habit), all users should be aware of them, because only the fastest emergency medical treatment can save a victim of a true overdose. There is little that nondoctors can do except keep the subject's head down, the limbs warm, and give artificial respiration if breathing stops. The main thing is to get help fast. Our laws against cocaine assure that the buyer almost never knows how much pure drug he is getting, so special caution is needed when taking the first hit of a buy.

Most people find that, when using cocaine as an erotic stimulant, an average 10-milligram line will do fine. Experienced users, especially if they have been snorting enough for tolerance to set in, often increase this to 15 milligrams or more and repeat it every hour or so. As the saying goes, drive at your own risk, for a cumulative toxicity does develop, varying with the individual, as well as irritation to the nasal membranes. That "line," by the way, is usually estimated as a little pile, $\frac{1}{2}''$ long by $\frac{1}{16}''$ wide by $\frac{1}{16}''$ high. The crystals should be chopped to a fine powder with a single-edge razor on a glass surface to spare the nose as much as possible. The membranes can be soothed with a nasal douche of warm, weak saltwater.

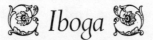

# Iboga

THE root bark of the equatorial African shrub *Tabernanthe iboga* is a drug that few Americans have ever heard of, unless they remember Hunter Thompson's charge that its alkaloid, ibogaine, was what Nixon's pixies slipped Edmund Muskie to make him cry on camera shortly before he lost the 1972 New Hampshire primary. Despite its obscurity, iboga was long ago placed on the

Drug Enforcement Agency's list of controlled substances, an example of preventive prohibition.

In Gabon, several tribes use iboga in rituals aimed at communication with their ancestors and in lion hunts that require men to stay alert but motionless for days. Ibogaine increases temperature, blood pressure, and glandular activity; its effects corroborate native use of the plant as an aphrodisiac and cure for impotence. There are reports from both Africa and the United States of frenzied passion continuing unabated for the better part (in fact, the best part) of a day after the participants ingested about a gram of the root. Unfortunately, iboga and ibogaine are among the hardest highs to find unless one has friends who travel in West Africa or work in pharmacological research labs.

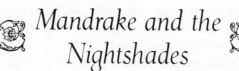

# Mandrake and the Nightshades

AT FIRST thought it may be hard to understand why these toxic plants are included in a book on aphrodisiacs. Anyone who has ever taken them and forgotten his lover's name will know that they are not something to be swigged every time you want to get it up. Still, they have been included in too many love philters to ignore. The *Ananga Ranga* suggests the juice of *bhuya kokali* (*Solanum jacquini*, a species of belladonna) mixed with ghee and sugar, for the amatory strength of ten men. Datura seeds are likewise added to ganja candies in India. The first-century Roman bucolic poet Columella calls mandrake *vesanus* (mad) because it was a noted ingredient of the strongest love potions, those which drove several of his contemporaries to insanity or death. Halfway across the world, Mexican Indians were adding small amounts of the related *tecomaxóchitl* (*Swartzia nitida*, or milk-cut chalice vine) to their *chocolatl*.

Such behavior is not easy to explain. Neither I nor any of my acquaintances who have tried these drugs, nor, as far as I know, anyone who has ever written of them, has ever described a true erotic experience under their influence. And yet the legend persists.

Most members of the nightshade family—including belladonna, datura, and mandrake, around which the dizzy tales collect—contain varying amounts of several anticholinergics, compounds that block the nerve transmitter acetylcholine. These chemicals—left- and right-handed forms of hyoscyamine (atropine) and scopolamine—disrupt the autonomic nervous system, which controls automatic life processes like heartbeat, breathing, and peristalsis. Atropine is mainly used today as a digestive-tract relaxant before surgery and as the best agent known for dilating the pupil of the eye—a fact that is reflected in the huge dark eyes of the Renaissance Italian beautiful woman (*bella donna*) who gave one of the nightshades its name. Depending on dosage and the exact amounts of each form of these molecules in the plant, the effects will extend further back along the nerves to eventually disrupt the acetylcholine pathways of the brain. When this happens to too great an extent, respiration ends and death begins.

In sublethal doses, nightshades are best described as deliriants. They may induce a comatose sleep, but usually this is preceded by intense and spasmodic physical excitation, tremors, excruciating dryness of all mucous membranes, and often true hallucinations, in which the subject vividly experiences something which can later be shown not to have happened.

The nightshades were associated with many of the early ecstatic religions of the Near East and Mediterranean, which centered around an experience of death and rebirth—the worship of Tammuz, Osiris, and Dionysus. Our most notable surviving document of this use is Euripides' play *Bacchae*, in which King

Pentheus, trying to suppress the cult, becomes the avatar of the dying god when he is dismembered by his own mother among the frenzied, wide-eyed maenads.

Nightshade use survived in the evolving remnants of these religions that became European witchcraft, and the confessions of witches abound with tales of midnight orgies, broomstick flights by externally applied ointments, and copulation with the cold hard tool of the Devil himself. We can surmise that Satan in this case was a dildo used ritually to fertilize the women and crops of the whole community in the name of the Horned God, but we cannot be sure which details were literally true and which were stories improvised to hide the truth from the Inquisitors or to get them to ease up on the thumbscrews.

As a group, humanity seems to be afflicted with the same amnesia about the aphrodisiac use of nightshades that the plants produce in individuals. The Biblical tale of Leah (Genesis 30:14–24), trading mandrakes for a night with her husband Jacob, so that his preferred wife, Rachel, could use them to end her sterility, no longer sounds plausible, even though it is said that Rachel gave birth to Joseph nine months later. We are left with a bizarre roster of superstition: mandrake was said to grow only under gallows from the ejaculated semen of hanged men. It was easy to find because it glowed in the dark, but you had to douse it quickly with a woman's urine or menses to keep it from running away. When uprooting it, you had to plug up your ears, then tie a dog to it and throw the cur some meat out of its reach so the animal would be killed by the screech of the root spirit instead of yourself.

Once in your possession the mandrake, especially if the root were forked so as to look human, would pump up your charisma, ward off evil, increase money left near it overnight, make Satan's angels get you any lover you wanted, find its way home if you lost it, and kill you if you overworked it—but it would only do so if you bathed it in milk or wine every Friday night, the day sacred to Aphrodite, who was known as Mandragoritis.

The only lead we have is that the nightshade alkaloids seem well suited for mental programming, from within or without. European police used scopolamine as a truth serum for years until it was shown that confessions were more what the interrogator wanted to hear than the truth itself. The Greeks called belladonna *Circeia* because they held it to be the herb with which Circe turned Odysseus's men into loyal swine. Even Charlie Manson didn't get a tight psychosexual grip on his acolytes until their regular acid tabs were supplemented with belladonna. One of the Family seems to have suffered a forty-point drop in IQ and corresponding rise in docility from the drug, according to Ed Sanders's documentation in *The Family*.

The nightshades can certainly paint real illusions. There was the recent case of a California dreamer, eager to experience the spirit world, who drank a thorn-apple (datura) tea in the woods and soon was blindly fleeing a host of demons and hobgoblins on bleeding feet. He attracted help only by accident, by lighting fires to keep the "voodoo people" at bay.

Nightshade hallucinations can fulfill fantasies acknowledged or unconscious, as the following anecdote will illustrate. This is one possible explanation why the spirit of deadly nightshade (belladonna) has so often been identified as a woman (at least by men) and why the nightshades have been considered aphrodisiacs.

Along with the hullabaloo over more publicized drugs, the mid-1960s also produced a minifad for belladonna, especially at eastern universities. To try out the rumored phantasmagoria, one acquaintance of a friend swallowed a large black capsule of the stuff before going to a party. Some time later, feeling uncomfortably warm, he took a few minutes' rest in the bathroom. When he looked in the mirror, he saw his face slashed to ribbons and bleeding hideously, but as he gasped and turned away, his eyes fell on a tub suddenly filled with more gore. Having had enough, he sought fresh air.

Outside, he felt better, especially when he met a beautiful

coed whom he'd been eyeing for weeks, also taking the air. They hit it off well and walked to his dorm with some mutual friends they met along the way. There the two snuggled up for a heart-to-heart that waxed more and more delirious till the cruel light of morning showed his worried roommate asking why he had been obliviously necking thin air half the night. The friends who had walked him home agreed that they knew the girl, but explained that she had been quite invisible as they'd walked to his building.

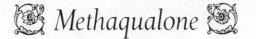

# Methaqualone

BETTER known as Quaaludes from the recently discontinued Rorer product, or 714s for the number stamped on the tablets, methaqualone is a hypnotic sedative little used in medicine but much used by a small but persistent public. Today methaqualone is about our sixth most popular drug, behind only alcohol, tobacco, coffee, cannabis, Valium, and possibly cocaine. When prescribed for sedation it is generally in a 75-milligram dose three times a day. Occasional dizziness, sweating, and a wicked hangover are the usual side effects. It may interfere with dreaming in REM sleep. Alcohol dangerously compounds its effects. With prolonged use tolerance builds, dosage increases, and withdrawal can bring on the same kind of convulsions as that from heroin.

It has acquired an unusual reputation as a "loosening up" aphrodisiac among people who take 714s illegally but less often than a prescription would call for. The tongue flaps and wobbles so easily that compulsive honesty can lead to embarrassing revelations. There is a tingly feeling in the skin, especially of fingers and toes. It's easier to fantasize. "The same sequence of word associations that might take ten minutes to drift toward the topic of sex in a normal conversation can happen in maybe a minute on ludes," explained a production man at a national magazine. Another told how, the day after selling some to three women who lived upstairs, he was accosted at their doorway on his next visit and ended up living with them for three months.

Both sexes agreed that methaqualone is more euphoric, or at least less dysfunctional, for women than for men. Men who take ludes regularly tend to have elevation problems. In more moderate use, the hypnotic loss of sensitivity may make climax control easier, but then there is less urge to hold back if the trigger is tripped.

One woman quipped that they're all right if you don't mind having your partner fall asleep in you. But the best that a Quaalude, or better, a half, can do is to lower the initial barriers, so that love the first time is as good as it would otherwise get only after you had known the person for a while.

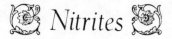 *Nitrites*

IN THIS case we refer not to the carcinogenic sodium and potassium nitrites used on bacon but primarily to amyl nitrite. This is a vasodilator and smooth-muscle relaxant sold by prescription to control heart spasms in angina pectoris. It is a volatile liquid whose fumes are inhaled after the glass ampules in which it is sold are broken open. For some years they have been a minor underground high, primarily among gays and swingers. Called poppers from the noise they make, amies yield a flash of only a few minutes, with a swooning sensation, a slowdown of time, a thumping heart, and giddy relaxation a bit like laughing gas. As muscle relaxants, poppers are good for opening the anal sphincter for cocks or hands, but they are best known for the way they prolong and intensify orgasm when sniffed just before climax. "It's as if I'm being shot into orbit when I come," said one user. "Each spurt feels like Old Faithful."

Amyl nitrite sales have increased steadily since the late 1960s, even though most physicians now use nitroglycerin for angina cases. But now the nonmedical nitrite market has expanded further with a dozen or more products called Rush, Locker Room, Essence of Man, Heart On, Jac Aroma, et cetera, sold through sex shops and by mail order. They are composed of a similar compound, butyl nitrite, and butyl alcohol. . Butyl is cheaper and easier to get than black-market amyl, and it has essentially the same effects. An even cheaper approximate substitute is ethyl nitrite, the sweet spirits of nitre still sold over-the-counter at some pharmacies despite its vanishing appeal as a household remedy.

There is little medical knowledge about the long-term effects of the nitrites, but a few whiffs once in a while seem to create no problems for many people. A significant number report bad headaches a few hours later, however, especially from the butyl forms. It is known that vasodilators can provoke migraines in those disposed to them. Nitrites are a perilous choice for anyone with low blood pressure; there is even a chance that suddenly lowered blood pressure could turn a latent aneurysm or other unrecognized circulatory problem into a life-threatening danger, but so far no deaths have been attributed to these compounds. Their hypotensive spinout lasts just two or three minutes, minimizing problems, but it can sometimes deflate a bone if pressure dips too low.

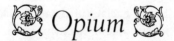 *Opium*

"I FELT like a human dynamo, fucking for over two hours with complete control over my orgasm. I could feel the sex energy building up in my gut and spreading through my whole body. I could have gone on all night, maybe forever, it felt. She must have had twenty orgasms. We were both delirious with love or lust or whatever it was. When I finally decided to come it was like an explosion of light."

The satisfied customer here quoted from Adam Gottlieb's *Sex Drugs and Aphrodisiacs* must sound to many as though he had made a mistake in the name of his potion. How can opium, the epitome of drowsy dreams, ever be such a tremendous turn-on?

Opium begins as the milky juice of the unripe seed capsules of the kind of poppy called *Papaver somniferum*. Once the petals have fallen, shallow slits are cut in the pods, and as the sap exudes it is collected and sun-dried until it becomes the soft black tar of commerce. This product contains up to 25 percent active alkaloids, mainly morphine, codeine, and the nonnarcotic muscle relaxant papaverine. Traces of more than twenty others are present.

Poppy extract is one of the oldest known drugs. The cut pods were found in the remains of Swiss villages on Lake Constance well before 2000 B.C. Known as "plant of joy" to the Sumerians, its use passed from Mesopotamia and Egypt to Greece and Rome, to Europe by way of the Arabian physicians who inspired Paracelsus. Opium smoking was not introduced into China until Emperor Ch'ung Ch'en outlawed tobacco in the seventeenth century and the British East India Company decided to expand its opium business by smuggling it into China. It did not become big business there until the British forced the trade on China in the Opium War. Knowledge of how to use the drug as an aphrodisiac seems to have developed more widely in China and India than in the West. The Chinese enclave at Batavia (Djakarta), for example, was famous for an opium electuary called *affion*, of which tales are told of wives fleeing their husbands after many hours of jousting had failed to break their lances.

Throughout its travels, opium has been known primarily for sleep, dreams and relief of mental and physical pain. In moderate to large amounts these effects predominate, but in smaller doses there is a mild stimulation of the spinal nerves that control pelvic blood flow and erection of both penis and clitoris, even while the rest of the body is becoming more relaxed. Small amounts of opium partly anesthetize the surface nerves of the glans (in both sexes) enough to bring their owner more control over release, but not enough to deaden the deeper layers. Opium can teach us to delay climax until the genital plexus is fully charged with neural energy, sexual tension is at its peak, and the orgasm can finally boil away in its full splendor. Once this lesson is learned with the artificial aid of opium, it can usually be repeated without the drug. Poppy gum can be a direct beginner's aid to the same kind of potential pelvic health and awareness as is the aim of Tantric yoga and such systems as Edward O'Relly's *Sexercises*. It is not a road that one can travel often, but it can open up virgin territory that can then be more reliably mapped by other methods. The similar discoveries that can be made through psychedelics, cannabis, or even a little extra oxygen, show that the joys are not direct results of the drug but are released by their aid from our locked closets.

One other quality helps turn a little black smoke into a long longing. Time slows. Peace descends. Bills vanish. Tension ebbs. The first exhalation after the sweet vapor takes hold is the foamy sigh of a wave sliding back into its companions over a warm sand beach. A fly may fly by. The breeze from its wings ruffles the hairlets on your arms; its buzz sends shivers up your spine like a lover's whisper, moist in the ear. Your legs may fall slightly open from the sudden relaxation, touching bare knee against bare knee. The microscopic silk and sandpaper of mingling skin lights the oven and puts solder on the tip of the iron. The bread starts to rise. Electricity paints the lips. Phosphorus burns in the groin. The tiniest contact expands to feel like a slow thigh moving up into the crotch. Skin, you both realize, flows over itself like quicksilver; limbs fit into each other's spaces as many ways as a thief's hand in the till. His head would nestle comfortably right here; there's room for her breasts there, and there. Arms and necks were meant for each other. Four legs are more economical than two. Living models of your bodies try all the postures of Aretino as you look into each other's mind's eyes, and you haven't even finished the pipe yet. Opium is one of the best unbridlers of fantasy ever discovered.

Naturally, some preparation must go into such a scene. It often doesn't work with total strangers. Comfortable surroundings and mutual attraction are essential for any magic to work. Even when the participants and conditions are right, the drug itself must be used very judiciously.

There are three main ways opium can be taken. The safest, because effects are more immediate and dose easier to control, is smoking. Actually it is not smoked but rather evaporated into the lungs by holding a flame *under* the pipe—use a long-stemmed metal one if you can't find a true opium pipe. One of the glass ones used for hash oil will do in a pinch. Drop a ⅛" pellet in the bowl and heat it until the white vapor begins to rise, then immediately inhale deeply and hold the breath for a few moments. Hold the pipe at an angle so the melted tar doesn't clog the pipe. Subjecting the opium directly to a flame is a great waste, as it will be burned and destroyed before much of it reaches the lungs.

Opium can also be eaten. About ¼ to ½ gram, a piece the size of a small pea (start with the smaller amount when first trying it), is simply sucked until it dissolves in the mouth, or it can be made into a tea with a bit of hot water. Though the smell is cloyingly sweet, the taste is bitter, and nausea often develops soon after swallowing because some of the morphine is converted by the stomach's hydrochloric acid into apomorphine, a strong emetic. Queasiness is less severe if the dose is swallowed gradually, over an hour's time.

Perhaps the best way to use opium as an aphrodisiac is to stick it up the ass. Nausea is avoided, effects are felt in an average of fifteen minutes instead of forty-five, as when eaten, and stimulation of pelvic nerves is more intense because the drug is absorbed nearby. When tension of vaginal muscles is a problem, the suppository can be an effective relaxant, and it is equally good for making sodomy easier and entry less painful. To administer, the bowels must be empty. Spread the *sides* of one finger with K-Y jelly or a similar lubricant (petroleum-based greases like mineral oil or Vaseline will hinder absorption), and place a small opium pea on the *tip* of the digit. Massage the anus a bit to relax the sphincter, then slowly and gently push the pellet as far in as you can. (Fist-fucking enthusiasts may be able to reach the large intestine, but a finger's length will do.) In women for whom vaginal penetration is normally painful, a pessary there or a cream made of opium mixed with K-Y or Noxzema has sometimes provided a breakthrough.

As with most good things, certain unpleasant facts about opium must be faced. First is the importance of not overdoing it. Do not succumb to the temptation of thinking the first dose was too small and some more will be just right. Wait till next time. Opium is seven times weaker than morphine and about forty-nine times weaker than pure heroin, but too much of it can still slow one to a standstill. If you or a friend have been overenthusiastic and you fear an overdose, *get a doctor fast.* Strong coffee will help in the meantime, as well as artificial respiration if the error was so bad that the breath is in danger of stopping. The amounts suggested here are safe, even for those who are very susceptible to the drug, but slightly more can defeat the amatory purpose and take you right to the dreamy torpor.

Nor can it be used often. Contrary to propaganda, a few pipes will not doom you to a life of pawning your mother's shoelaces, but tolerance will often start to develop after a few days, certainly after a few weeks. The sexual disinterest and even genital atrophy among opiate addicts is well known, and even several days of indulgence markedly lowers resistance to colds and other infections.

Finally, the poppy's natural dangers have been compounded by artificial ones Possession of any amount is a felony in most states, and many judges show more leniency to baby rapers. Because opium is a rare luxury here, narcotics agents do not sell it to their victims as often as heroin, cocaine, or cannabis, but it is still terribly unwise to buy it from anyone you don't know personally. Never has there been a market in which caveat emptor is better advice.

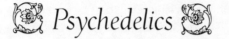 *Psychedelics*

AT FIRST, using LSD as an aphrodisiac may seem like using a fire hose as a water pick. The initiate is overwhelmed by one of the most complete learning experiences known to humanity, and there is often no thought of watching *only* the erotic film while simultaneously seeing every movie in town.

LSD and the other psychedelics have fairly nonspecific effects, that is, they release experiences that are already latent in the nervous system and which can sometimes be triggered by other methods, such as long practice of yoga. Common to the experiences is what is called dissolution of the ego. Perhaps it's better described as a spreading of this normally restricted part of consciousness to include unconscious needs and desires, unnoticed floods of sensory input, the relationship of the personality to all other beings in the web of life, the panorama of evolutionary history, the taste of childhood, and the evidence that energy is solid and all matter is dancing energy, ad infinitum. Naturally, in any culture that has insisted on suppressing sexual enjoyment as long as ours, much of what gets released will have to do with sex. And since a good case can be made for the sexiness of the ultimate push-pull, yang-yin ground of being, this is only proper.

Though the universe may be sexy, the tripper may not feel that way, especially when the experience is still new—there is just too much going on at once. Personal or interpersonal problems may present themselves in terrifying detail to be worked out first. This is where a guide, experienced with acid but not high at the time, is crucial, for with a few deftly reassuring suggestions, road-blocks can in a few minutes dissolve as the shadows they are. We have not the space for detailed instructions on the use of this force. Too many excellent manuals have been written, and undue condensation can be dangerous.

LSD may be cited as a case in which the antidrug laws have "worked." After the major suppliers of quality acid were busted in the late 1960s and early 1970s, many people gave it up or never tried it rather than take their chances with the sloppily made stuff that then became the norm. Judging from the product exported from California in 1978 however, we may be in for a revival.

During acid's first heyday, Dr. Timothy Leary made one of his many big splashes by saying in a 1966 *Playboy* interview that LSD was the greatest aphrodisiac in the world and that from its plateau a few hours of tender fucking can give a woman several *hundred* orgasms, while the man climbs to the top of the exploding mountain with exquisite endurance and control. To those who were more accustomed to Dr. Alfred Kinsey's reported average of one and a half minutes between intromission and emission, Leary's statement must have seemed fantasy and boast. To those more in tune with their own possibilities and LSD's, his words were a clue to development. And to certain adepts of Tantric yoga the news was no news.

LSD is an erotodelic—it can enhance the act of love by slowing down the mind and widening its focus. A full dose of acid typically abolishes the sense of time, making it pointless to rush toward orgasm, as if it too were going to be illegal in a few minutes. There is time for tenderness, and the intermelting of bodies continues even without movement. I don't know of anyone who has felt compelled to count spasms in that situation, but I have no doubt that for some women Leary's figure could be literally true. Others would much rather just break down in happy tears a few climaxes short of that nongoal.

Other psychedelics can be mental aphrodisiacs in slightly different ways. MDA (methylenedioxyamphetamine) keeps its late 1960s nickname of "love drug" because of the way its point of view helps lovers read each other's minds. Peyote, in a similar way, can help diagnose the ills of a relationship as few other plants can.

Then there are the harmal alkaloids. Including harmine, harmaline, harmalol, and tetrahydroharmine, they grow in Syrian rue (*Peganum harmala*), the western Asian bean caper (*Zygophyllum fabago*), passionflower (*Passiflora incarnata*), and most abundantly in the Amazonian visionary vine called *yagé* or ayahuasca (*Banisteriopsis caapi*).

In Egypt the oil pressed from the seeds of Syrian rue is sold as the aphrodisiac hallucinogen *zit-el-harmel*. Yagé in small doses is used among Brazilian Indians as an erotic stimulant during puberty rites and other occasions. In full strength it is an extremely potent and tricky hallucinogen whose full use requires a five-year apprenticeship to a *yagero* qualified to teach the ins and outs of astral travel, divination, and clairvoyance with the plant.

Harmal compounds have been little explored by Western psychopharmacology. It is known that the typical cup of yagé contains about 400 milligrams of them, and pure harmine can produce a psychedelic experience when absorbed through the mucous membrane under the tongue. Researchers have seen increased sexual activity in rats given several of the substances, and many theorize that they interact somehow with a related compound (6–methoxytetrahydroharmane) found in the pineal body and said to accumulate in this "third eye" with the development of yogic or spiritual powers.

# 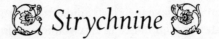 Strychnine

OH, THE heartless mockery of reality! The spirit of vegetation conjured up what should have been the perfect aphrodisiac tonic, but carelessly made it too poisonous to use. The major alkaloid of the *Strychnos nux-vomica* tree, strychnine is a stimulant of both motor and sensory nerves, especially in the lower spine. It increases the acuity of all five senses, so much so that a touch, a sound, or a flash of light is enough to throw the sufferer into the violent convulsions of overdose, similar to those of tetanus. All muscles are taut, strongest predominating; the back may be so arched that only feet and head touch the floor. Strychnine, and to a lesser extent its close relative, brucine, are cumulative poisons. When taken repeatedly, any amount above the tiniest doses (½ to 4 grains of the seeds) soon passes from tonic to toxic.

Strychnine has found many people willing to brave its dangers. It was in the white man's medicine bag from 1750 to recently. Under the names *kuchala* or *vishtinduk*, it is still much used in India, where it is native to the Coromandel (southeastern coast). It also grows in Sri Lanka, Southeast Asia, and the East Indies. In these areas, and for a time in the West, strychnine found favor as a bitter digestive tonic and remedy for chronic constipation. Ayurvedic medicine holds it in store as a powerful tonic for long-term debility, but *no tonic effects have ever been confirmed in any dose whatsoever.*

As an aphrodisiac strychnine often was and occasionally still is combined in Mexico and the southwestern United States with damiana, a similar but infinitely less perilous tonic from the same area. In Asia, ground nux vomica seeds have long been added to hashish-based sex potions, a practice responsible for occasional fatal ecstasies over the centuries.

In Europe strychnine was combined with goldenseal and ergotine, or with iron, quinine, and chloroform. Sometimes, doctors merely had patients make their own fluid extract by pouring a pint of boiling water over an ounce of nux vomica seeds and taking a daily dose of 1 to 3 drops.

Today's standard antidotes for a strychnine overdose are diazepam (Valium), barbiturates and/or mephenesin, combined with an emetic or stomach pump as soon as possible. Amyl nitrite is sometimes recommended because of its rapid effect of lowering the blood pressure in the midst of convulsions. I mention these remedies only on the off chance that a reader would be so foolish as to try nux vomica without a doctor's guidance. Both individual tolerance and the potency of the seeds vary widely. Hence, I cannot emphasize too strongly that this is *not* a drug for personal experimentation, no matter what level of frustration or curiosity exists.

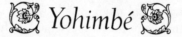

# Yohimbé

THIS tropical West African tree yields one of the few aphrodisiacs that have been tested in Western medicine. The official conclusion as stated by Louis Goodman and Alfred Gilman (*The Pharmacological Basis of Therapeutics*) is that there is "no convincing evidence" for a directly erotic effect. The reddish brown inner bark from *Corynanthe yohimbe* has been available to doctors for treatment of impotence since the early 1930s, at which time Norman Douglas crowned it "the most effective of modern provocatives." It is one of the precious few potions that may excite a genuine undeniable horniness within an hour, as opposed to a gradual tonic effect over days or weeks, but because there are many people for whom it does nothing, it cannot reach the highest pinnacle of the definition.

For years yohimbé enjoyed great repute until hormone therapy for impotence came of age, and veterinarians formerly used it on laggard bulls and stallions. It has even begun to replace Spanish fly in love-potion jokes—like the one in which a young man dining with his date calls the waiter aside, slips him a packet of yohimbé pills, and asks him to have the cook put one in the soup. Dinner is long delayed, and an embarrassed waiter finally whispers that the chef dropped in all the pills by mistake and is waiting for the noodles to lie down.

Yohimbé contains numerous alkaloids. Ajmaline (or rauwolfine), ajmalicine (or δ-yohimbine), and corynanthidine (or α- or iso-yohimbine) are all also found in Indian snakeroot (*Rauwolfia serpentina*) and seem to have similar hypotensive (blood-pressure-lowering) effects. The most abundant and active ingredient is yohimbine (alias quebrachine, corynine, or aphrodine), also found in the bark of the South American quebracho ("ax-breaker") tree.

Yohimbine is extracted as a white powder which can be dissolved under the tongue, snorted, or ingested by capsule in doses of 5 to 20 milligrams.

There is no consistently noticeable difference between the actions of pure yohimbine and the crude bark. Yohimbine penetrates the brain well and can produce increased pulse and blood pressure, sweating, physical restlessness, urine retention, or sometimes nausea. Sexual excitement may result from stimulation of nerves in the sacral plexus, inducing hyperemia (engorgement with blood) of the pelvic area. Spontaneous erections that sometimes pop up without outside enticement are guaranteed to promote a grateful respect for herbs even among the most skeptical.

The yohimbé alkaloids also have a blocking effect on the neurotransmitters acetylcholine and epinephrine, which is presumed to cause the herb's mild psychedelic effects, especially in larger doses of up to 50 milligrams of yohimbine. The mental changes run toward heightened empathy and emotional openness rather than the visual fireworks and confrontation with the ultimate more characteristic of full doses of LSD or psilocybin. Skin sensitivity is sometimes enhanced so much that the specific ecstasy of flesh flowing and bodies melting into each other is often felt for the first time.

Yohimbé is a weak serotonin inhibitor. Part of its aphrodisiac effect may be a reduction of accumulations of this vasoconstrictor in some persons. An excess is known to produce increased blood pressure, sleepiness, lack of energy, and loss of interest in sex. The increased flow of blood to the genitals can be harmful in some cases of impotence caused by inflammatory disease, such as prostatitis.

All users must note the fact that yohimbé is a monoamine oxidase (MAO) inhibitor. This means that it blocks the enzyme that normally protects the body against certain amines, such as the tyramine widespread in foods, which can otherwise cause a dangerous rise or fall in blood pressure, associated with cardiac problems, headaches, and in severe cases, even death. As a result, the widespread tribal custom of fasting before a sacrament is advisable, and yohimbé is, despite its pleasures, not a substance one can use regularly or casually.

It should not be taken with other drugs, especially not with other MAO inhibitors. Most tranquilizers must be avoided, although Librium (chlordiazepoxide) or sodium amobarbital can be safely used if the yohimbé voyager develops an anxiety reaction. Tryptamine and harmal alkaloids, most sedatives, antihistamines, amphetamines and all diet pills, mescaline, alcohol in any form, cocoa, aged cheese, pineapples, bananas, sauerkraut, and any other foods rich in the amino acid tyrosine (converted to tyramine in the body) must also be avoided on the day yohimbé is used. Don't forget to consider prescribed medication, as many are long-acting MAO inhibitors, and merely stopping their use for a day or two will not avoid the danger. Finally, any persons with diabetes, hypoglycemia, or any organic problems of liver, heart, kidneys, or circulatory system should avoid yohimbé altogether.

Yohimbé is one of the best-selling items on the "legal highs" counter of the reviving herbal market, but few of the companies that sell it include such a list of precautions. Companies like Woodley Herber include it with many other herbs in herbal smoking blends, some intended for the I-couldn't-score-any-pot-today market, others resting primarily on yohimbé's laurels. Yohimbine, tried for a time by doctors as a local anesthetic, is sold under names like Yocaine as a cocaine substitute. As such it is a less energizing but more directly aphrodisiac sniffable; it takes effect in a few short minutes and eliminates the nausea that the oral route sometimes entails in the entrails. Here again, there are no MAO warnings on the labels. Most yohimbé experimenters survive this ignorance without damage, but there have been a few close calls of users hospitalized with near-fatal hypotension. Many take too small a dose to do much of anything, and if they feel dizzy or headachy, often just give up on this particular herb.

To experience the rewards of yohimbé without its dangers, avoid the foods listed above on the day of use.

> Simmer 3–6 teaspoons of the powdered bark (up to 8 if in shaved form) in a pint of water for 10 minutes. As with all psychoactives, it is best to start with a low dose, even at the risk of no effect, and work upward—especially if you are a person of low bodyweight. As the tea cools, dissolve 1 gram (1,000 milligrams) of vitamin C in the cup.

California self-experimenters proved that the yohimbine ascorbate thus formed is more easily assimilated. Sip the drink slowly, preferably with honey for your taste buds' sake. Because of the vitamin, the first effect—usually a warm, shivery feeling in the lower back—will be felt in about fifteen minutes instead of thirty to forty-five minutes. The experience seldom lasts more than three hours, and there are no after effects except the fatigue that normally follows an intense experience.

At best, yohimbé should be thought of as a sort of botanical sex therapist. The preparation and precautions make it too cumbersome to do regularly, even if one wanted to subject oneself to a psychedelic every day or so. For some men, the external boost in the rigidity department provides the confidence needed to relax into natural sexual response more completely than ever before, a benefit that can then accrue to every encounter thereafter. Except for the spinal stimulation, the yohimbé experience is much like low doses of the more common psychedelics. Like them, it can be used to warm up special holidays in bed or to make sure your id remembers the fullest possibilities of orgasm, wherein *all* the tension is released, the beauteous present is momentarily eternal, and all the colored wheels fly away in the brain.

# PART IV

# *Enlarging the Menu*

# 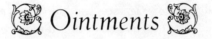 Ointments

THE search for male aphrodisiacs reveals an undercurrent of thinly veiled rage against the man's most fickle and sometimes embarrassing organ. If it fails to gather into itself the heat needed to stoke a waiting furnace, then by God let's blister it with enough heat to last for weeks. Love lore lists scores of inflammatory ointments, some made with a touch of forgiveness, some downright infernal.

Most men have through time avoided the need for these concoctions, but the demand for them has never entirely disappeared. Perhaps the impulse is dimly related to pubertal circumcision rites, meant to imbue young men with a sense of the pain of life. The Australian aborigines sliced open the urethra along the whole length of the penis, and some Arab tribes flayed all the skin off of it—fatally about one-third of the time. But if the son so much as gasped, he was unworthy, disavowed, cast out. These horrors must have led to a certain amount of impotence, which could surely be remedied by a little more blood on, or from, the sword. A little pepper juice might even have felt soothing to some of these wounded spears.

The idea behind most of the salves was what we now call hyperemia—skin irritation, heat, and engorgement with blood near the surface. Oil of wintergreen is an old favorite which can be tested in a jiffy by rubbing some Ben-Gay on the sucker. In *The Perfumed Garden* the Shaykh Nefzawi suggests a mild one: chewing a few cardamom pods and rubbing the aromatic saliva on the glans. The Chinese, when making a rice flour poultice of cubeb peppers, usually add some mallow roots to mitigate the sting.

Avicenna mentions the spit trick with cubebs instead of cardamom and suggests a little honey with ginger and pepper or with the virulent irritant scammony. Nicolas Venette lists a venerable recipe of honey, storax, clarified butter, and goose fat as binders; ambergris and musk for fragrance; and spurge, ginger, pepper, and chives for bite. In fairness to both doctors it must be said that they caution against careless use of these and record them mainly as curios.

An occasionally used prescription of Dr. William J. Robinson was a weak mixture of camphor, oil of cayenne, and mustard oil in petroleum jelly. This showed up slightly altered as a London patent medicine of the mid-1940s, whose effect reminded many of napalm, even the women who were subjected to it secondhand.

Some unguents were made for use on the scrotum, to increase sperm production and output of "the spiritous humor or fluid which renders a man robust, hearty, and courageous," as Galen presciently described testosterone. A mild example of the testicle plasters was: cinnamon, gillyflower, ginger, and theriac* in rosewater and red wine, mixed with bread crumbs to make a paste.

The adventurous reader who decides to try any of these recipes should have on hand some A and D ointment or aloe vera gel. For an authentic historical touch, an ointment made from the soothing resin of a Middle Eastern evergreen, balm of Gilead (or

---

* Theriac was the meat of a poisonous viper, used in countless medicines as a supposed antidote to snakebite.

Judea or Mecca), can be applied to sore members in the aftermath of the hot creams.

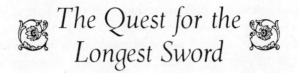

# The Quest for the Longest Sword

ARE you one of the thousands of men afraid to look a woman in the eye because your dick only puts out a measly ten inches? Well, weep no more, my friend. Gathered here on the convenient sheets are the worthless secrets of the ancient masters, a few that may effect some prodigy, some words on inflating or constricting your counterpart's parts, and certain measurements to help set you straight.

Most books that mention penis size begin with the anthropological statement that a long one is a powerful symbol of dominance among men and other primates, then tell us that size is of no consequence whatever in finding a mate or making love to her. This halfhearted reassurance is bound to fail when, as is usually the case, no hint of average measurements is given and the nervous reader is left to hold his own against fearsome imaginary studs parading their two-foot prongs.

Two areas of the body remain relatively unknown—the brain and the genitals—but explorers of the nether regions must also cope with ages of misinformation and fear. In earlier societies where the generative force was worshiped, people had a pretty good idea what to expect when somebody opened a toga, but fig leaves and whispers produced fears of inadequacy that are still, after "sexual revolution," a fine cause of impotence. Just how universal this nervousness is in the developed nations was shown a few years ago when CIA records about an early-1960s plan surfaced. Operation Penis Envy would have involved dropping cases of enormous condoms over Russian cities, the packages prominently labeled EXTRA SMALL. The hoax was allegedly never perpetrated, but do you think the Soviets would have let on if it had been?

Less comical results of ignorance regularly appear in the letters columns of sex magazines, where terrified men admit to being literally on the verge of nervous breakdown or suicide because they feel their perfectly normal organs are somehow puny or misshapen. Hence a few hard facts are in order before we speak of improvements. Medical surveys show that 75 percent of all erect penises are between 5″ and 7″ long; the average is 6″. Another 20 percent are within an inch either way of this range. Slightly more than 3 percent are between 8″ and 9″, while less than 1 percent are larger than 9″ or shorter than 4″. Concerning possible racial or national differences, there is much contradictory folklore but no reliable information.

For the vast majority of men, the only reasons to undergo the risks of penis-enlarging schemes are macho bravado or idle curiosity. Some women, but perhaps not even a majority, seek the ultimate schlong as a sort of sexual avocation, just as many men are fascinated by big breasts, but very few of either sex count measurements among their major excitements.

Nevertheless, even a man who got the short end of the stick can satisfy all but the biggest women because of the vagina's wonderful elasticity. It is *almost* true that "one size fits all." And any number of strap-on extenders can be had to adapt an average sword to even the biggest scabbard, although from the standpoint of male sensation, this is a poor solution to a vexing problem.

For those who dare to put their personal puds on the line, there is no lack of gadgets and recipes. For example, the medieval Arab doctor-philosopher Avicenna says:

> It is increased in size by rubbing in hot fats and oils
> after friction with a rough cloth and the pouring of dif-

ferent sorts of milk over it, mostly sheep's milk; and by the subsequent application of a pitch-plaster, to draw the blood. . . .

But I think the prize must go to the eggplant plaster invented by the Guyanese. To make it one cuts an eggplant in half lengthwise and scrapes a long channel in the central pulp. The victim then makes a paste of *bois bandé* (or *babandi*, "tightening wood," the root bark of a tree, which may contain a weaker cousin of strychnine called brucine), the heads of 6 to 12 old-fashioned phosphorus matches, 2 or 3 *zozos* (hot pimentos), a dozen each of peppercorns and cloves, and 1 or 2 vanilla beans. This fiery mud is spread on the cavity of the halved eggplant, which is then closed and bound around the penis, with the foreskin drawn back, for eight to ten hours. The flames are then doused with soapsuds and lukewarm mallow water. The seared pecker, allegedly a size larger, becomes erect at the least touch and ready for "almost painful" copulation for some time thereafter.

Among the painless alternatives is basil. There is a long tradition among Italian men that this fragrant herb can increase size. There is no apparent reason why and no tests have been made to prove or disprove the belief, but at least the medicine is tasty and harmless even in huge amounts.

Finally there are various types of physical stimulation. In ancient China a physician named Wu Hsien devised the following ritual for "sharpening the tool," from the book *The Tao of Love and Sex*, to be done between midnight and noon, while meditating in peace and facing east, with neither a full nor empty stomach and after breathing deeply forty-nine times:

> Then he should rub his palms together until they are hot as fire. Next he uses his right hand holding his scrotum and his *yü hêng* [jade stem]; his left hand rubs his abdomen beneath the navel in the round and round manner, turning left for eighty-one times, and then he uses his right hand rubbing the same spot in the same

manner, except turning right for another eighty-one times. Then he stretches his right hand and lifts his *yü hêng* from its root, swinging and shaking it left and right, hitting both legs numerous times. Then he hugs his woman and gently thrusts his *yü hêng* into her house of Yin, nurtures it with his woman's secretions and breathes in his woman's breath [it was believed that woman's breath nourished the male, and vice versa]. After this he should use his palms rubbing his jade peak in the manner of making a thread from fibres uncountable times.

The last few years have been the growth of a sizable market for contraptions to take all the manual labor out of Wu Hsien's method, without bothering with the niceties of breathing and alignment. "Peter pumps" or "penis exercisers" cost from twenty to two hundred dollars. Most are a simple vacuum pump with various latex or plastic sheaths. Some, like the Chartham Method device from England, come with a booklet outlining a system of exercises, hot baths and massages supposed to make the increase permanent.

The whole idea is to get more blood into the cavernous spaces of the organ. Some physicians have stated that these machines may cause fibrous degeneration of the erectile tissue if the pressure is too strong, but I have seen no estimates of how much the average penis can stand before damage sets in. Nor have I heard anyone explain how these expensive gimmicks differ from balling tried-and-true Rosie Palm and her five sisters.

At present, the longer-dong market is but a trifling offshoot of the breast-development biz, which reaps millions from silicone implants, suction pumps, and glorified exercise books. Both are masculine rackets; no such business grew up around vagina-tightening, although women have long used herbs for the purpose. *Geranium maculatum*, found throughout the Northern Hemisphere as American cranesbill root, European wild alum, or Indian kino root, is perhaps the best known, in a solution of 1 teaspoon powdered root to ½ pint water.

Masturbation was credited in some Victorian medical books and many parents' warnings with reducing the size of the penis, if not making it fall off. Most sexologists since van de Velde have admitted that masturbation tends to enlarge the clitoris, so there is some reason to believe that it may do the same for the male counterpart.

The modern medical consensus is that usually there is nothing that will turn a Vienna sausage into a kielbasa. Don't bother wearing baggy pants so as not to impede circulation. Hormone therapy brings some results in cases of arrested development, but the best general advice to those who want a larger hose is—use it. In fact, size changes seem most easily made before adulthood, so the best way to ensure full genital growth at maturity is sexual freedom during childhood and adolescence.

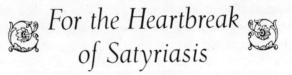

# For the Heartbreak of Satyriasis

*If as you lie on your couch after a meal you are
excited by the alluring train of sensual desires,
then seize the shield of faith.*
—SAINT JEROME

ONE of the strangest brief encounters of my life was the experience of watching a truck driver's face, contorted with rage, as he drove past my lover and me picnicking near a park roadway, screaming the worst insult he could think of: "Lovers!"

Until brought up short by some such fiasco, the seeker after elixirs is optimistic at first. One encounters the names of so many that the whole earth seems awash with them, drenched in them, choked as by weeds. Every morsel taken into the mouth must be tainted with the stain of delight. But soon it's obvious that not all that's advertised is gold. Many so-called aphrodisiacs have no effect at all. Even worse are the unreliable ones, which may put one partner to sleep while the other languishes on a fiery mattress. Even without aid, Aphrodite herself is at times a bit too obstreperous, as when one is sick, tired, or in the mood to be alone. There are times when each of us needs a coolant in the system. I have not intentionally tested any of those mentioned herein except toil and abstruse pursuits, but I can assure you that these two work very well.

Certain jobs are chastity prone. The question of whether priests should have the best sex or no sex at all has been a hot one all through history, and probably before it. The "abominations" in the temples were one of the main reasons the Mosaic Jews gave for massacring some of the tribes they dispossessed. The Greeks and Romans allowed many forms of sexuality into their religions, but even among them the vestals were chaste and the priests of Attis had to give up the gonads. Custom required the severed organs to be flung into the first house the novitiate passed as he ran streaming down the street. The same sacrifice was required for membership, or dismemberment, in the bizarre Russian sect called the Eunuchs (*Skoptsi*), which surfaced in the eighteenth century. Believing that Adam and Eve were literally created sexless, the Eunuchs mutilated each other at their meetings. The rule was relaxed to allow a child or two before gelding—to replenish the roster.

Most celibate faiths let priests keep their equipment as long as they promise not to use it. The highest spiritual progress has been supposed to stem from complete denial of bodily concerns. "Even a sick monk uses only cold water, and to take anything cooked is wanton luxury," explains Saint Jerome in the desert.

"Let your companions be women pale and thin with fasting."
Sackcloth, exhaustion, as little sleep as possible, were their pleasures. "To induce you to take baths, they will speak of dirt with
disgust." Even then the fight was hard:

> Yet that same I, who for fear of hell condemned myself
> to such a prison, I, the comrade of scorpions and wild
> beasts, was there, watching the maidens in their dances:
> my face haggard with fasting, my mind burnt with de-
> sire in my frigid body, and the fires of lust alone leapt
> before a man prematurely dead. . . .

A similar tradition has unflowered in the East, where chastity
is the first vow of the *bramacharya*. One of the few men who has
tried it both ways and written about it, Aleister Crowley, found no
difference in his thoughts or work, only in his enjoyment. Still,
many are the platonists who hold that intercourse has no importance in a relationship of total communication. Among yoga postures, the *siddhasana*—a sitting position in which one heel is
pressed against the perineum and the other against the groin
above the genitals—is especially recommended for quieting desire's fires.

Vegetarianism, gluttony, fasting, feasting, and boozing can
do nicely. Long fasts usually calm libido, but a short one may
strengthen it. Try a watery, bland, acid diet with lots of weak tea,
vinegar, cucumbers, lemonade, gooseberries, watercress, and lettuce. Vegetarianism may not work because it has definite health
benefits for many people, but it can be calming. Dick Gregory
says he and his wife have successfully tried sexual fasting to learn
about lust: "I got tired of looking at women as, so to speak, meat.
I wanted to clear my mind. . . ."

Try plenty of hard work, anxiety, or endless study. Isaac
Newton supposedly escaped Aphrodite altogether. When Jean
Jacques Rousseau failed a Venetian harlot, she told him, "Give
up the ladies, Jean, and take up mathematics." When the rabbis
of ancient Israel decreed how often each class could screw, they

allowed peasants one a week, merchants one a month, sailors two a year, and scholars one every two years.

When King Phillippe of France, in one of Boccaccio's tales, hears of the beauty of the Marchioness of Monferrato, he decides to visit her in the Marquis's absence. Her reality so surpasses his courtier's picture that his desire is transparent. That night, in the presence of her court and friends, she serves him a banquet fit for a royal guest. Partway through, though, the king realizes that every course is made of chicken, hens only. Then turning to her merrily, he asked, "Madam, are hens only born in these parts, without ever a cock?" Taking the occasion to set him limp, she replied, "Nay, my lord, but women, albeit in apparel and dignities they may differ somewhat from others, are nevertheless all of the same fashion here as elsewhere." Neither he nor the other guests could mistake her drift, and his highness doused his unwelcome fire.

Some truly ingenious customs have been invented to prevent arousal. There's the ordinary cold shower; there's the chastity belt, and there are plates of lead hung all over the body, by which Pliny says Roman doctors cured the orator Calvas, who had such a hair trigger he came at the mere sight of a pretty woman. Though it wasn't necessarily invented for the purpose, the Venetian congress, which judged marital quarrels by watching the pair copulate, must have been a superb passion-killer.

Among the herbs and drugs, camphor is supposed to be lust's worst enemy, long sniffed and chewed by monks, but from the outside at least acting like other rubefacients. Agnus castus, called Abraham's balm or the chaste tree, was a great favorite of the *nyet* set. Then there are black willow leaves, lady's slipper, purslane, hemlock poultices, hellebore, juice of fresh vervain or asphodel root, valerian, Rocky Mountain grape root, and hawkweed (*Hieracium*). Medieval nuns grew the parthenium flower while their brethren made a wine of rue. Both unsexes took two-week treatments of a drink made from white water-lily roots (*Nym-*

*phaea alba*) and opium poppy syrup. According to Pliny, forty days of nymphaea water will make a man permanently sterile. These days heroin addicts are just as well known for complete disinterest in sex, but antihypertensive drugs or lots of laxatives seem to work almost as well.

A coffee habit is a good one to cultivate as an anaphrodisiac. A queen of Persia once wondered why her grooms were going to such trouble to tie down a stallion for gelding when they could just feed it coffee every day instead. Likewise an English surgeon named Abernathy once said, "Any man that drinks coffee and soda water, and smokes cigars, may lie with my wife."

Tobacco is another good passion-killer. There is a well-established statistical correlation between tobacco smoking and impotence, lowered sperm and testosterone counts, and sterility. This may be due to the inhibition of testosterone production by carbon monoxide in the blood, as well as lowered oxygen supply. Hasn't done much for the taste of kisses, either.

The would-be saint should stay out of the sun, for it seems that turning the light down low may actually be *un*romantic. Study of the pineal gland indicates that it produces an "antisex" hormone, which regulates desire cycles. Production of this inner wet blanket is inhibited by light, as has been shown in experiments with rats and surveys of Eskimos, who make love less when the sun dips below the horizon.

Still horny? Maybe magic will work. Emeralds touched to the genitals cool them. So do lynx ashes in wine, a turtledove's heart in a wolfskin pouch, and dried frog powder. In Roman times, one of the strongest love repellents was believed to be a little of the beloved's blood.

Tried everything? Still getting results? Have some bacon. Nitrites used to preserve it are essentially the same as the potassium nitrate (as well as bromides) which once were, and may still be, dished out to prisoners, soldiers, and students at military and religious academies. But the second greatest anaphrodisiac of all, age, was the butt of the old joke in which one gray-haired old soldier says to another: "Remember the saltpeter they gave us in the war to quiet us down? Well, it's just beginning to work."

The best one of all? Satiety—lots of messin' around. If it only worked longer. . . .

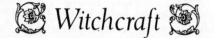 # Witchcraft

> The moon is nothing
> But a circumambulatory aphrodisiac
> Divinely subsidized to provoke the world
> Into a rising birth rate.
> —CHRISTOPHER FRY, from
> *The Lady's Not for Burning*

TO THE Neolithic farmers who went two by two into their fields to sow wild oats by moonlight, it was love that sanctified the planting, fertilized mother earth, and called down torrents of semen from sky father. This belief is the basis of popular religion and witchcraft throughout most of the world. In some parts of Christian Europe, procreative gods were disguised as phallic saints, such as Saint Foutin of Provence, saints Guignolet, Regnaud, and Gilles. In Medieval France the stone penis of Saint Greluchon was scraped and the powder drunk by women for fertility. The spring carnival procession of a huge wooden phallus called *Il Santo Membro* was not abolished in the Neapolitan town of Trani until the eighteenth century.

The rituals for crop renewal usually seemed to work, just as those for hunting had worked twenty thousand years before. Naturally, other sympathetic acts were devised to restore potency or attract a lover by imitating the result in symbol. The harvested lust-grown grain was baked in cakes and breads shaped like genitalia, anciently offered back to the gods, later reserved more and more for the objects of human affection. The Greeks had their *mylloi*, the Romans their *coliphia* and *siligone*, sold by bakers and courtesans. In the Middle Ages, a woman who wanted a certain man would give him cockle bread, with or without his knowledge. The loaf was kneaded on her buttocks. It often had a dash of menstrual blood and was baked in a small oven placed on a board over the nude woman's hips. One needs to burn to light a fire.

The birds and animals thought most amorous were sometimes made into potions. Turtledove, baked in an oven till dry and crisp, then powdered and added to the intended's wine, was an old favorite. A Hindu recipe used a kite in the same way, while in Medieval Europe the ashes of a weasel were applied to a man's big toe while he was sleeping to gain his love.

It is well known that many charms depend on a material connection with their target, such as hair or fingernail clippings. A Persian Muslim recipe for increasing a husband's love requires that one of his shirts be taken, and boiled in a basin of rosewater along with cloves, cinnamon, cardamom, and a piece of parchment with his name and the names of four angels written on it. All the while, the practitioner is to read the Yasin chapter of the Koran backwards seven times.

Mayan women used the following rite to make a man come back "like a docile domestic animal." On the night of the moon, in a *cenote* (a pool inside a cave), the "patient" bathes. She is adorned with plumeria (*Thulunhuy*) flowers, and around her dancers joined in a spiral make nine turns in each direction, singing *kay nicté*, the song of the flower. The "patient" takes home the flowers and some of the water to be cooked into food for her errant lover.

Ordinary enticements are invested with added power by making them more elaborate. Elongating the eyelashes with mascara is not usually thought of as witchcraft today, but it was in India when one had to make an attractant mascara by gathering certain herbs and burning them on the wick of a lamp of oil and blue vitriol (copper sulfate). A man was sure to put more than usual eloquence into his flute if he was first required to anoint his reed with the juices of seven rare hand-gathered herbs: *bahupadika, Tabernamontana coronaria, Costus speciosus, Pinus deodora, Euphorbia antiquorum, vajra,* and *kantaka.*

Portentous orotundity is often intended to bamboozle the intended. The *marejoa* (love prayer) of the Guarauna in the Orinoco basin is such, only used after all other remedies have failed to win the woman a man loves. Through a mutual friend he announces the start of the marejoa, so she may tremble. A shack of *temiche* palms and *cazubo* leaves is built within earshot of her house. According to A. Turrado Moreno's *"Etnografica de los indios guaraúnos"*:

> The client, the *brujo* [shaman], and a clown gather at the hut. The brujo makes a very long cigar and inhales a great deal of smoke. He puffs the smoke toward the woman's house, then begins the marejoa chant, melancholy, monotonous, mysterious, which ended, the brujo, coming out of his hiding place, scatters toward her house bits of *yuruma* meal [the dried pitch of a certain palm].

The clown then told the girl that the deed had been done, and she often, for fear of death, succumbed right on cue.

Certain rituals tried to harness the fixity of death directly to the constancy of love. The Celtic "dead strip" was done by cutting a strip of skin from a corpse dead nine days and tying it around the beloved's wrist or ankle while he or she was asleep, then removing it before morning. As might be imagined, the force of the charm, and the affair itself, might be broken if the sleeper awoke during the operation.

A number of curses were invented to confer impotence or sterility on an enemy. Some are like the trick of bubble gum or funny signs on the back of the kid chosen Nerd for a Day. One of the most feared of these was a bit of mouse shit smeared on the sleeve or rump of the unwary. The people of central Sumatra believe in sperm applied to a woman's clothing or body as a powerful tie.

The natives of the island of Dobu in the western Pacific have carried magic to its logical conclusion. According to the Dobuans, sexual desire and copulation exist only because men and women are constantly working magic on each other. An extensive repertoire of ritual is part of the community's heritage, but they also feel that a man or woman is not fully alive unless he or she has devised secret personal spells. The function elsewhere filled by a specialist is on Dobu everybody's business.

Most modern, forward-looking materialists dismiss the entire subject as superstitious nonsense—until they are faced with the choice of walking under or around a ladder. What we now call the "scientific reasons" for an herb's effect—the action of its alkaloids on the chemistry of body and brain—is still "magical" to those who know no pharmacology. Most magical rituals demand a certain amount of effort, a certain specificity—like the one that directs a man to anoint his penis with the lard of a *medium-sized* goat. Most try to draw the spirit of the lover or sorcerer out of the body to act upon the spirit of the target. Though psychic science is in its infancy, its experiments have convinced most skeptics who care to look that mental energy can indeed be focused for material effects. Most of us still call a process magic because we don't understand it—love, for instance.

Love magic certainly has an edge in groups where everyone believes. Imagine the pretty young woman, getting ready for bed, noticing a glittering dab of dried semen on her instep and suddenly remembering how assiduously one of her swains tied her sandal that day. Imagine her finding a tiny square cut from the inside of a bodice she had hung near her window the night before. How could she confront anyone with such insubstantial evidence? How could she help but sigh and reflect on the devotion and ingenuity her lover has shown. The charm has already begun its work.

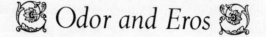# Odor and Eros

BEGINNING on May 11, 1988, the United States will be crazy with aphrodisiacs, according to the noted psychic Criswell. A person or persons unknown will inflame whole cities with sex stimulants in water supplies and air conditioning systems. Millions will make love in streets and fields, overcome by fragrant clouds of an airborne elixir, possibly escaping like radioactive gas from aphrodisiac research centers. Florida will become the first entirely nudist state, and high government officials will be caught with their pants down. Discovery and mandatory distribution of an antidote will get things back to dismal normalcy by March 30, 1989.

If this charming episode ever comes to pass, it will probably result from research on *sexones*—chemical agents of subliminal sexual communication thought to function in humans much like the extensive repertoire of such compounds in mammals and insects. In nonhumans these odors are called *pheromones* ("transferers of excitement") to indicate that they serve many causes besides sex. They are used as signals to announce food or danger, as personal identity tags so mothers and young can find each other, as trail or territory markers, as indicators of rank among social animals, and as threat signals to induce fear in an enemy.

Systems of five or ten pheromones are the dominant mode of communication among many species, especially social insects and nocturnal animals such as mice, who must avoid noise and visibility to escape predators. They often override all other senses. Pheromone researchers like to tell of incidents like the male tortoise seen trying to mount a head of lettuce over which a female had recently walked.

A specific pheromone stimulates reciprocal grooming in ants. So strong is its message that a dead ant is often groomed for several days until the decay odor prompts the others to carry it to the rubbish pile. Conversely, a live ant coated with death scent by scientists will be thrown away again and again, no matter how often it rejoins the colony.

Pheromones are incredibly strong, as are the noses that smell them. It takes 500,000 female gypsy moths to yield .02 gram of gyplure, the pheromone isolated by U.S. Department of Agriculture scientists to attract males to traps and control the pest. Each male will respond to fewer than a hundred molecules, and each female produces enough to attract a billion males. Muskone, the active principle of musk, is one of the most powerful scents known. A tiny amount can fill a huge room in minutes, but a gram of it in the open air would lose only one percent of its weight in a million years. Dogs are able to detect the odor of one human fingerprint on a glass slide exposed to the weather for a week. Even humans, with one-fortieth the olfactory area of dogs, can smell one 460-billionth of a gram of ethyl mercaptan (odor of rotting meat).

Chemical sending and receiving is apparently the oldest form of communication. University of Michigan researchers have studied *Streptococcus faecalis,* an inhabitant of the human intestine and one of many bacteria that exchange DNA in a form of protosexual reproduction called conjugation. In each encounter, one "male" bacterium passes a gene bundle (plasmid) to a "female" who has enticed "him" by secreting a chemical attractant. After the plasmid transfer, the former female becomes a male, and the former male acquires the ability to secrete the attractant as a female.

But what relevance does all this have to humans? This question is the subject of heated debate. Some scientists argue that sight, sound and touch dominate our reactions completely and that, while humans have scent glands and receptors, they are vestigial organs with little effect on our sex lives. This view is supported by the work of David Goldfoot of the Wisconsin Regional

Primate Research Center. Studying copulins (vaginal scents) in rhesus monkeys, Goldfoot concluded that they have no direct effect on mating and that learning and individual mood are much more important in monkeys and all higher primates. Advocates of this side point out the primate lack of a *vomeronasal*, or *Jacobson's*, *organ*—a large supplementary smelling center at the base of the nasal septum with ducts opening into the mouth.

On the other side of the argument is a large, diverse body of evidence, from both folklore and science, which suggests that scent is a strong unconscious force in every sexual reaction we have:

>•— Richard P. Michael, discoverer of rhesus copulins, believes they *do* modulate passion in the monkeys. Copulin levels vary with estrogen secretion in the menstrual cycle, and, when transferred from a normal female to one without ovaries, they stimulate the normal male response. In fact, *human* vaginal secretions turn on monkey males almost as well.

>•— History records numerous cases of Shunammitism, the rejuvenation of the aged by young people of the opposite sex, without intercourse. The name comes from Abishag the Shunammite, a young maiden given to old King David (I Kings 1:1–4). Likewise the Roman L. Clodius Hermippus lived to the age of 115 by surrounding himself with the exhalations of young virgins. (The ancient worldwide custom of nose kissing rests on a similar belief in the value of inhaling the breath of the opposite sex. Even today Sanskrit uses the same word [*ghra*] for "smell" and "kiss." The Persian *bujal* equates "smell" and "love," while the French *sentir* means both "to smell" and "to feel." Based on scents from another source, a venerable European belief recommends an apple

or a handkerchief rubbed in the armpit as an irresistible love token.)

🌿— Biologist Lewis Thomas in *The Lives of a Cell* reported the experience of a British scientist who lived alone on an island. When the man collected and weighed the daily clippings from his electric shaver, he found that his beard grew much faster when he went to the mainland and encountered women.

🌿— If human scent signals are not functional, it is strange that we give off so many of them. *Apocrine* glands in our armpits and around our nipples secrete their characteristic odor, while a slightly different one emanates from glands near the genitals and anus. Still others grow on the face and feet. All of them are activated at puberty. Dr. Alex Comfort classifies smegma as a scent as well as a lubricant, similar to boar taint, and suggests that circumcision is a case of repression of sexual odors. Furthermore, each race has its own pattern of scent, as though the trait were an evolutionary device to keep sexual attraction within the population group. Caucasids have a strong, meaty smell. Negrids, with more glands on the torso, give off more ammonia. Mongolids, with the fewest scent glands and the least body hair, tend to a faint fishy odor. Australids have a large concentration of glands near the anus. And all racial groups have a tradition of being offended by the body odor of the others.

🌿— Humans are not so smell-blind as is generally believed. Several experiments have shown that subjects can usually identify their own clothing from that of others by smell alone. Another test found that most people can pick out a piece of paper which had been stepped on by a bare foot and learn to identify different people (even twins on different diets) by the smell of their hands.

᚛— The nose is a sex organ. It grows along with the genitals at puberty and has erectile tissue similar to the penis or clitoris, which engorges with blood during arousal. Loss of the sense of smell from chemotherapy, x-ray exposure, or accident is often followed by loss of interest in sex. And olfactory sensitivity in women, especially to musklike odors, has been shown to vary with estrogen levels and thus diminish drastically in pregnancy.

᚛— Current knowledge about brain structure suggests that the nose is the shortest route to the nerve centers that control sexual behavior. The reproductive centers in the hypothalamus and the limbic septum, as well as the feeding and fighting centers of the amygdala, are both right next door to the olfactory bulb, and all are in the deepest, most ancient part of the cerebrum.

᚛— In the early 1970s Martha McClintock, at Harvard, and Michael Russell, a California researcher, proved that when women live together for a long time, their menstrual cycles tend to synchronize. Russell, using the underarm secretions of a colleague who did not shave her armpits and had a regular 28-day menstrual cycle, proved that the synchronicity effect is caused by scent by daubing "essence of Genevieve" on the upper lips of sixteen women volunteers. Since the same effect occurs in mice, the possibility arises that other rodent reactions have their equivalent in human females, too—such as the normalization of estrus by the hormones in the urine of male cage-mates and spontaneous abortion from the scent of an alien male introduced into the cage.

If human sexuality does depend so heavily on sexones, there remains the problem of why we so diligently mask them with the perfumes of plants and other animals, with all the jasmine, civet, ambergris, and strawberry sprays. To this there is no easy answer, for it is the same as asking why we so often repress our sexuality.

Psychologists Irving Bieber and Michael Kalogerakis think

that the sexual orientation toward the opposite gender at ages two to five involves an attraction to the opposite-sex parent's body odor and a corresponding repulsion from that of the same sex. They further suggest that the odor attraction is driven into the unconscious by the incest taboo, leaving the conscious field wide open to surrogates, which may include perfumes and the odor of such fetishes as feet, leather, urine, hair, or latex. Others feel the denial of human sexones stems from the need of a society's leaders to control the sexual energy of the group, hence the prestige attached to rare fragrances and the "lower class" disgrace of body odor.

Whatever the reason, there is no such thing as chemical rape in humans. Janet Hopson, whose *Scent Signals* brings an admirable order to this smelly chaos, gives sexones a purely subliminal role to the dominant visual and emotional modes of sexual attraction. The evidence, she says, points to a preliminary check for odor compatibility before the other factors operate, and an unconscious addition or subtraction of desire from other turn-ons, a sort of fine tuning of desire.

One thing is sure: If the human sexone(s) are ever isolated and bottled, there will be plenty of customers. Perfumiers are in the forefront of research but keep their results strictly secret. Auto makers would love a more powerful sales scent to replace the "new car essence" they spray on their vinyl interiors. Politicians would put a dab on their handbills. It would have important medical applications—contraceptive nasal sprays that would use smaller amounts of hormones than the pill; detection of diseases by body scent; olfactory treatment of impotence and frigidity; and perhaps detection of ovulation by smell for a fail-safe rhythm method.

Meanwhile, there is no need to wait for the experts before exploring the powers of sexones for oneself. For the nasally inhibited, a simple resolve to sniff without preconceived judgments of foul and sweet can open up a whole new world of sensation.

# 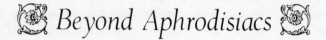 Beyond Aphrodisiacs

EVEN if we grant all the miraculous powers of all the miraculous elixirs of folklore, there are some things that no aphrodisiac can do. Not one can suddenly abolish the big hairy wen on the chin, the roll of fat around your mate's midriff. Not one can mask dull conversation, blame throwing, nagging, leaving the refrigerator door open, or whatever else irks you most about the stranger you were madly in love with a few months ago. Some say real love is not blown by such imperfections, and any lack of response is really stunted emotions in the beholder. This explanation should be tried, as it assumes reality is kind, and removes a load of guilt from one of the aggrieved parties in many a sexual fiasco. But, as Diotima once told Socrates, love is neither good nor beautiful, but only a yearning for same. Aphrodisiacs can increase the force of desire, but no potion can change its course.

Eros cannot be domesticated—only won, asked for, found, or given. As for sustaining love in another, imagination is the truest aphrodisiac; like a faceted gem it constantly glints with unexpected lights, and the "same old face" looks like an exciting new affair. Without it, even novelty goes stale, and the champagne loses its bubbles.

Some erotic herbs and drugs can help dissolve the inhibitions that result from being made to feel guilty about sex as a child, but no potion can give the shy one courage to lay that old ego on the line with the first hello. Nor can it teach what to say after that. The sparkle in the eye begins in the head, and without the right words, that first zero-gravity tumble into conversation will bumble to a halt, all the smoldering gazes wasted. The art of being subtle without disguising one's intentions is a fine one, an art for which there are no textbooks. Take a tip from Dr. Ernest Dichter, who began the modern age of advertising in 1941 with a study for Pontiac on the imagery of pistons.

No aphrodisiac but practice can give a person the empathy and timing needed to fan the flame in another without blowing it out. In general, as Balzac noted, intimacy moves from a distich to a quatrain, to a sonnet, to a ballad, to an ode, to a cantata, to a dithyramb, and anyone "who begins with the dithyramb is a fool." But if the audience hearing those sweet songs is already swooning in the aisle, additional verses can lead to a rush for the exit.

Whatever elixirs and blandishments you choose, take heart from the work of Dr. Paul Cameron at the University of Louisville. Dr. Cameron took the trouble of charting the thoughts of 3,146 people to find out that erotic ideas cross the mind of the average person under thirty every ten minutes (and last for fifteen, if my own research is reliable). Even in his 70- and 80-year-old subjects, Cameron found fantasies occurring once an hour.

If we assume eight hours of sleep and then compare "every ten minutes" with Kinsey's national average of 2.46593 copulations per week, we find an astounding unused erotic potential of 669.53407 occasions every week. So don't worry if you run out of aphrodisiacs; within the human head is an endless supply.

# Appendix:
## 🌺 Major American 🌺
## Herb Suppliers

CALIFORNIA

Electric Earth Herbs, Box 261, Sonora, Cal. 95370
Herb Products Co., 11012 Magnolia Blvd., N. Hollywood, Cal. 91601
Herbal Holding Co., Box 5854, Sherman Oaks, Cal. 91413
Herbs of Mexico, 3859 Whittier Blvd., Los Angeles, Cal. 90023
Home Grown Herbs, Box 1697, Modesto, Cal. 95354
Lhasa Karnak Herb Co., 2513 Telegraph Ave., Berkeley, Cal. 94704
Magic Garden Herb Co., Box 332, Fairfax, Cal. 94930
Nature's Herb Co., 281 Ellis St., San Francisco, Cal. 94102

CONNECTICUT

Capriland's Herb Farm, Silver St., Coventry, Conn. 06238
Natural Resources, 25 Chestnut St., Danbury, Conn. 06810

ILLINOIS

Dr. Michael's Herb Products, 1223 N. Milwaukee Ave., Chicago, Ill.
60622

## INDIANA

Indiana Botanic Gardens, Inc., Hammond, Ind. 46325

## KENTUCKY

L. S. Dinkelspiel Co., 229 E. Market St., Louisville, Ky. 40202

## MICHIGAN

Harvest Health, Inc., 1944 Eastern Ave. SE, Grand Rapids, Mich. 49507

Woodley Herber, Box 172, Okemos, Mich. 48864

## MISSOURI

Luyties Pharmacal Co., 4200 Laclede Ave., St. Louis, Mo. 63108

## NEW JERSEY

Givaudan, 100 Delawanna Ave., Clifton N.J. 07014 (fragrance specialists)

Rocky Hollow Herb Farm, Box 215, Lake Wallkill Rd., Sussex, N.J. 07461

## NEW YORK

Aphrodisia, 28 Carmine St., New York, N.Y. 10014
Franklin Pharmacy, 764 Franklin Ave., Brooklyn, N.Y. 11238
Kiehl's Pharmacy, 109 Third Ave., New York, N.Y. 10003
Magickal Childe, 35 W. 19 St., New York, N.Y. 10011
Milan Laboratory, 57 Spring St., New York, N.Y. 10012

## NORTH CAROLINA

Carolina Biological Supply House, 2700 York Rd., Burlington, N.C. 27215

## OREGON

Nichols Garden Nursery, 1190 Old Salem Rd. NE, Albany, Ore. 97321

Haussmann's Pharmacy, 6th and Girard Ave., Philadelphia, Pa. 19127
Penn Herb Co., 603 N. 2nd St., Philadelphia, Pa. 19147
Tatra Herb Co., 222 Grove St., Morrisville, Pa. 19067

RHODE ISLAND

Greene Herb Garden, Greene, R.I. 02827
Meadowbrook Herb Garden, Route 138, Wyoming, R.I. 02898

SOUTH CAROLINA

Columbia Organic Chemicals, 912 Drake St., Columbia, S.C. 29209

TEXAS

Paracelsus, Inc., 1217 N. Collins, Arlington, Texas 76011
Swamp Fox Herbs, Box 66133, Houston, Texas 77006

VERMONT

Vermont Country Store, Weston, Vt. 05161

WASHINGTON

Real Concept, Box 30593, Seattle, Wash., 98103

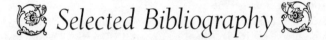 *Selected Bibliography*

Airola, Paavo O. *Sex and Nutrition.* New York: Award Books, 1970.

Apicius. *The Roman Cookery Book.* Translated by B. Flower and E. Rosenbaum. London: George G. Harrap, 1958.

Ashe, Penelope. *The Naked Chef: An Aphrodisiac Cookbook.* Port Washington, N.Y.: Ashley Books, 1971.

Beck, Bodog, and Smedley, Dorée. *Honey & Your Health.* Revised edition, 1944. New York: Bantam Books, 1971. Reprint.

Bernay, L. *Les Aphrodisiaques: Pour ou contre le doping sexuel?* Paris: Editions de Gerfaut, 1968.

Bieler, Henry G. *Food Is Your Best Medicine.* New York: Random House, 1965.

Bloch, Iwan. *Odoratus Sexualis.* 1934. New York: AMS Press, 1976. Reprint.

Bosch, Vernon. *Sexual Dimensions: The Fact and Fiction of Genital Size.* Dayton, Ohio: Ax Produxions, 1970.

Brillat-Savarin, Jean Anthelme. *The Physiology of Taste, or Meditations on Transcendental Gastronomy.* Translated by M.F.K. Fisher. New York: Harcourt Brace Jovanovich, 1978.

Carrington, Charles (under pseudonym Dr. Jacobus). *Untrodden Fields of Anthropology.* New York: Falstaff Press, 1937.

Center for Science in the Public Interest. "Changes in Food Consumption Patterns by Americans Since 1910." Washington, D.C.: CSPI.

Chang, Jolan. *The Tao of Love and Sex.* New York: E.P. Dutton, 1977.

Clarke, Borden (ed.). *The Lucayos Cook Book 1660–90.* Morrisburg, Ont.: Old Authors Farm, 1959. Private printing.

Connell, Charles. *Aphrodisiacs in Your Garden.* New York: Award Books, 1966.

Crane, Eva. *Honey: A Comprehensive Survey.* New York: Crane, Russak, 1975.

Culling, Louis T. *A Manual of Sex Magick.* St. Paul, Minn.: Llewellyn Publications, 1971.

Davenport, John. *Aphrodisiacs and Anti-aphrodisiacs.* 1869. Reprinted in *Aphrodisiacs and Love Stimulants,* edited by A. H. Walton. New York: Lyle Stuart, 1966.

Dioscorides, Pedanius, *The Greek Herbal of Dioscorides.* Translated by John Goodyer (1655), edited by Robert T. Gunther. Oxford: Oxford University Press, 1934.

Douglas, Norman. *Paneros: Some Words on Aphrodisiacs and the Like.* London: Chatto and Windus, 1931.

———, ed. *Venus in the Kitchen.* Introduction by Graham Greene. London: Heinemann, 1952.

Dumas, Alexandre, père. *Dictionary of Cuisine.* Edited and abridged by Louis Colman. New York: Simon & Schuster, 1958.

Frascone, Jon Paul, and David, Mark Allen. *Aphrodisiac Cook Book: Meals to Pep Up Your Love Life.* Hollywood, Calif.: Ermine Publishers, 1975.

Frazier, Greg and Beverly. *Aphrodisiac Cookery: Ancient and Modern.* San Francisco: Troubador Press, 1970.

Gifford, Jr., Edward S. *The Charms of Love.* Garden City, N.Y.: Doubleday, 1962.

Goodman, Louis S., and Gilman, Alfred. *The Pharmacological Basis of Therapeutics,* fifth edition. New York: MacMillan, 1975.

Gottlieb, Adam. *Sex Drugs and Aphrodisiacs.* San Francisco: The 20th Century Alchemist/High Times/Level Press, 1974.

Grieve, Mrs. M. *A Modern Herbal.* 1931. New York: Dover, 1971. Reprint.

Haines, Paul. "A Critique of Pure Bawdry." *The Modern Thinker,* v. III, p. 290, 1933.

Harris, Lloyd J. *The Book of Garlic*. San Francisco: Panjandrum Press, 1974. Distributed by Holt, Rinehart & Winston.

Heartman, Charles F. *Cuisine de l'Amour: Aphrodisiac Culinary Manual*. New Orleans: The Gourmets' Company, 1942. Reprint (undated) distributed by Burt Franklin, New York.

Hendrickson, Robert. *Lewd Food: The Complete Guide to Aphrodisiac Edibles*. Radnor, Pa.: Chilton, 1974.

Henriques, Fernando. *Love in Action: The Sociology of Sex*. New York: E. P. Dutton, 1960.

———. *Stews and Strumpets* (volume I of *Prostitution and Society*). London: MacGibbon and Lee, 1961.

Hirschfeld, Magnus, and Linsert, Richard. *Liebesmittel*. Berlin: Man Verlag, 1930.

Hopson, Janet L. *Scent Signals: The Silent Language of Sex*. New York: William Morrow, 1979.

Hurwood, Bernhardt J. *The Whole Sex Catalogue*. New York: Pinnacle Books, 1975.

International Institute for the Study of Human Reproduction. *Biorhythms and Human Reproduction*. New York: John Wiley, 1974.

Kalyanamalla. *Ananga Ranga*. Translated by F. F. Arbuthnot and Richard F. Burton as *The Hindu Art of Love*. New York, Lancer Books, 1964.

Keys, John D. *Chinese Herbs: Their Botany, Chemistry and Pharmacodynamics*. Rutland, Vt.: Charles E. Tuttle, 1976.

Lappé, Frances Moore. *Diet for a Small Planet* (revised). New York: Ballantine, 1975.

Legman, Gershon. *Rationale of the Dirty Joke*. New York: Grove Press, 1968.

Lehmann, Friedrich R. *Rezepte der Liebesmittel*. Heidenheim, Germany: Erich Hoffmann Verlag, 1955.

Lewis, Walter H., and Elvin-Lewis, Memory P. F. *Medical Botany: Plants Affecting Man's Health*. New York: John Wiley, 1977.

Lust, John. *The Herb Book*. New York: Bantam Books, 1974.

Mann, Thaddeus. *The Biochemistry of Semen*. New York: John Wiley, 1954.

Mathison, Richard R. *The Eternal Search: The Story of Man and His Drugs*. New York: G. P. Putnam's, 1958.

Murat, Felix. *Bee Pollen: Miracle Food.* Miami, Fla.: R. Murat Co., undated.

Nefzawi, Shaykh. *The Perfumed Garden.* Translated by Sir Richard F. Burton. New York: Castle Books, 1964.

Niemoller, A. F. *Aphrodisiacs and Antiaphrodisiacs.* Girard, Kans.: Haldeman-Julius, 19—.

Null, Gary, and Null, Steve. *Protein for Vegetarians.* New York: Pyramid Books, 1974.

Passwater, Richard. *Supernutrition.* New York: Dial Press, 1975.

Petersen, Fritz. *Sex Food.* New York? 196— (8 pp.).

Pfeiffer, Carl C. *Mental and Elemental Nutrients.* New Canaan, Conn.: Keats, 1975.

————. *Updated Fact/Book on Zinc and Other Micro-Nutrients.* New Canaan, Conn.: Keats, 1978.

Pullar, Philippa. *Consuming Passions: Being an Historic Inquiry into Certain English Appetites.* Boston: Little, Brown, 1970.

Rinzler, Carol Ann. *The Book of Chocolate.* New York: St. Martin's, 1977.

Robinson, William Josephus. *America's Sex and Marriage Problems.* New York: Eugenic Pub. Co., 1928.

Rompini, Omero. *La Cucina dell'Amore.* Catania: Libreria Tirelli di F. Guaitolini, 1926.

Rouet, Marcel. *Le paradis sexuel des aphrodisiaques.* Paris: Productions de Paris, 1971.

Sailland, Maurice Edmond. *La table et l'amour; nouveau traité des excitants modernes.* Paris: La Clé d'Or, 1950.

Sandler, Merton, and Gessa, G. L. (eds.). *Sexual Behavior: Pharmacology and Biochemistry.* New York, Raven Press, 1975.

Silver, Jules (ed.). *Liebesrezepte aus der Geheimküche Amors.* Ghent: Ariston Verlag, 1975.

Steinmetz, E. F. *Kava-Kava: Famous Drug Plant of the South Sea Islands.* 1960. San Francisco: The 20th Century Alchemist/High Times/Level Press, 1973.

Turner, Nicholas. *Aphrodisiacs: Food for Love.* London: Latimer New Dimensions, 1975.

Tyler, Varro E., et al. *Pharmacognosy* (7th ed.). Philadelphia: Lea and Febiger, 1976.

United Nations, Food and Agriculture Organisation, Food Policy and
Food Science Service, Nutrition Division. *Amino-Acid Content of
Foods and Biological Data on Proteins.* Rome: United Nations, 1970.

United States Department of Agriculture. *Handbook of the Nutritional
Contents of Foods.* Edited by Bernice Watt and Annabel Merril. New
York: Dover, 1975. Reprint of USDA Agriculture Handbook #8,
*Composition of Foods,* 1963.

Vatsyayana. *Kama Sutra.* Translated by Sir Richard Burton and F. F.
Arbuthnot. New York: G. P. Putnam's, 1963.

Walton, Alan Hull. *Aphrodisiacs (Love Potions) from Legend to Prescription.* 1956. New York: Paperback Library, 1963. Reprint.

Wason, Betty. *Cooks, Gluttons and Gourmets: A History of Cookery.*
Garden City, N.Y.: Doubleday, 1962.

Wedeck, Harry Ezekiel. *Dictionary of Aphrodisiacs.* New York: Philosophical Library, 1961.

———. *Love Potions Through the Ages: A Study of Amatory Devices
and Mores.* New York: Philosophical Library, 1963.

Williams, Roger J. *Physicians' Handbook of Nutritional Science.*
Springfield, Ill.: Charles C. Thomas, 1975.

Wilson, Robert Anton. *Sex & Drugs: A Journey Beyond Limits.* Chicago: Playboy Press, 1973.

ABOUT THE AUTHOR

GARY SELDEN is the former science editor for *High Times* magazine. He is presently at work on a book that will draw the sexes
closer together. He lives with his wife in Queens, where there are
no distractions.